Clinical Tuberculosis

Second Edition

Sir John Crofton KB MD(Camb) FRCPEd and Lond
Professor Emeritus of Respiratory Diseases and Tuberculosis,
University of Edinburgh

Norman Horne MB ChB FRCPEd
Formerly Consultant Physician, Chest Unit, City Hospital,
Edinburgh

The late
Fred Miller MD FRCP DCH
Formerly Honorary Physician, The Children's Department,
Royal Victoria Infirmary, Newcastle upon Tyne

Sponsored by the International Union Against Tuberculosis and
Lung Disease and by TALC (Teaching Aids at Low Cost)

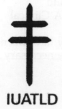

IUATLD

MACMILLAN

TALC

First edition 1992
Reprinted twice
ELBS edition 1994
Second edition 1999
Published by
MACMILLAN EDUCATION LTD
London and Oxford
Companies and representatives throughout the world

ISBN 0–333–72430–5

11	10	9	8	7	6	5	4	3	2
08	07	06	05	04	03	02	01	00	99

This book is printed on paper suitable for recycling and made from fully managed and sustained forest sources.

Printed in Malaysia

A catalogue record for this book is available from the British Library.

Acknowledgements

The authors and publishers wish to thank the following for permission to use copyright material:
Aids International for Table   from D J Girling, 'Adverse effects of anti-tuberculosis drugs', *Drugs*, 23 (1982) 56-74;
Churchill Livingstone for Figure 17 from F J W Miller, *Tuberculosis in Children*, New Delhi, Churchill Livingstone (1986);
World Health Organization for Table 13, Table 16 from WHO data and information; and for adapted material in Chapter 5 from 'TB/HIV: A Clinical Manual', Geneva, WHO (1996);
Every effort has been made to trace the copyright holders but if any have been inadvertently overlooked the publishers will be pleased to make the necessary arrangement at the first opportunity.

The Authors

Sir John Crofton became Professor of Respiratory Diseases and Tuberculosis at Edinburgh University in 1952. He has been Chairman of the International Union Against Tuberculosis and Lung Disease's tuberculosis treatment and tuberculosis diagnostic scientific committees, and a member of WHO's Consultative Panel on TB. He has lectured and advised in over 50 countries.

Norman Horne was President, Europe Region, of the International Union Against Tuberculosis and Lung Disease from 1982 to 1988, and has been Chairman of the Chest Heart and Stroke Association of Scotland since 1982. Formerly he was President of the British Thoracic Association, and WHO Visiting Professor in Medicine, Baroda, India.

Fred Miller was a consultant paediatrician and undertook many assignments for WHO, chiefly in India. He also wrote the book *Tuberculosis in Children* (Churchill Livingstone, 1982).

Contents

Foreword to First Edition

The International Union Against Tuberculosis and Lung Disease welcomes *Clinical Tuberculosis* with interest, gratitude and pride.

Interest, because clinical aspects are part and parcel of the essential knowledge necessary both to those dealing with the individual and those dealing with the community.

Gratitude, because precisely this type of manual for non-specialised practitioners and public health field workers was long and badly needed.

Pride, because the book is the result of the collaborative effort of two long-standing highly respected members of the Union, and a paediatrician, all of them with an immense experience with tuberculosis patients as well as with the problems and needs at national and international levels. The book bears witness to their indefatigable drive in trying to impart useful know-how to their colleagues and fellow workers striving under difficult conditions.

We now possess well established methods for prevention, diagnosis and treatment of tuberculosis as well as the concept of National Tuberculosis Programmes; the latter provide the system through which the effective means can be delivered.

Recent studies have re-awakened our awareness as to the magnitude of the problem: tuberculosis remains the biggest killer in the world as a single pathogen; while it hits children as well as elderly, the worst affected are adults between 15 and 59 years of age i.e. the parents, workers and leaders in society. Tuberculosis accounts for 26 per cent of all avoidable deaths in Third World countries.

The tremendous toll of tuberculosis is increasing in many countries due to the interaction of HIV and tuberculosis infections. However tuberculosis remains curable even in the HIV infected. The present remobilisation against the ancient scourge tuberculosis will, hopefully, be able to curb the present flaring up of incidence.

Moreover cost–benefit analyses have shown that short-course chemotherapy of tuberculosis, within the framework of national programmes, is one of the cheapest of all health interventions, comparable in cost to immunization for measles or to oral rehydration therapy for diarrhoea.

Those who fight tuberculosis, this inseparable but terrible companion of man, will find this comprehensive and clear book a mighty ally to assist them accomplish their mission with more competence, more understanding and more humanity, and will bring closer the time when proper diagnosis and adequate management of cases will stop the perpetuation of the disease, thus paving the way to its elimination.

Annik Rouillon, MD, MPH
Executive Director,
International Union Against Tuberculosis
and Lung Disease

Preface to the Second Edition

Professor David Morley, the Honorary Director of Teaching Aids at Low Cost (TALC), originally asked the authors to write this book for non-specialist doctors and health professionals in countries with a high prevalence of tuberculosis. We found it a fascinating challenge to try to produce a book in simple language which could be useful to workers who might have very few resources. The book was to be primarily about clinical tuberculosis. But we felt that clinical tuberculosis should be put in a framework of a National Tuberculosis Control Programme. Only in that framework could the mass of patients be effectively diagnosed and cured. Only in that framework could mass cure lead to mass prevention.

We had hoped that at least some doctors and health professionals in some countries would find the book useful. In the event it does seem to have met a real need. The demand has exceeded our wildest expectations. We initially arranged for French, Spanish and Portuguese translations, so as to make it available to the appropriate countries in Africa and America. But we have been delighted to find that many countries have wished to produce editions in their own languages. As we write (1997) it has appeared in fourteen languages, with editions in four others in various stages of preparation. Besides the languages already mentioned there are editions in Russian, Italian, Croatian, Chinese, Mongolian, Thai, Vietnamese, Arabic, Farsi (Iran) and Turkish. We are expecting future editions in Romanian, Indonesian, Urdu and Bengali. We are most grateful to the translators, publishers and distributors of all these editions. A preliminary estimate is that more than 70,000 copies in the various languages have been distributed in 125 countries. The book has been used by the World Health Organization and the International Union Against Tuberculosis and Lung Disease, and we hope by others, for their training courses.

In producing our first edition we had much help from a series of international experts. These included Professors John Biddulph (Papua New Guinea) and David Morley (TALC and UK); Drs Andrew Cassels (UK), Keith Edwards (Papua New Guinea), A.D. Harries (UK and Malawi), Wendy Holmes (Zimbabwe and Australia), Kanwar K. Kaul (India), A. Kochi (WHO), Colin McDougall (UK), S.J. Nkinda (Ethiopia),

Knut Ovreberg (Norway and IUATLD), S.P. Pamra (India), C.A. Pearson (UK and Nigeria), Annik Rouillon (France and IUATLD), Sergio Spinaci (WHO), Karel Styblo (Netherlands and IUATLD), H.G. ten Dam (WHO), Yan Bi-Ya (China). Once more we record our gratitude to them.

In preparing this second edition we have benefited from much discussion with international experts, notably those from WHO and IUATLD. In particular we thank Dr Hans Rieder of IUATLD who re-read our first edition in detail and made many helpful suggestions which we have incorporated.

The major changes in the present edition are in the chapters on HIV and tuberculosis and in the sections on chemotherapy. Since the first edition there is now much more experience of HIV. We have greatly expanded that chapter. In doing so we have utilised extensively the WHO publication *TB/HIV. A Clinical Manual* by Drs A.D. Harries and D. Maher (1996). We are most grateful to Dr Harries for constructive criticism of a draft of our chapter.

We have revised the sections on chemotherapy to make sure that they are consistent with the second (1997) edition of WHO's *Treatment of Tuberculosis. Guidelines for National Programmes*. We have also revised the Appendix on tuberculin testing in the light of recent recommendations by the International Union Against Tuberculosis and Lung Disease and informal discussions with WHO staff.

Much work has been done in recent years on 'molecular' aspects of tuberculosis. The detection of specific components of tubercle bacilli may ultimately lead to rapid diagnosis of disease and to rapid detection of drug resistance. Genetic classification of sub-strains of bacilli can already identify sources of local outbreaks. But none of the new methods is so far sufficiently simple, reliable and cheap for general use in poorer countries. So we have not included any details. The search continues for new drugs but none has yet proved sufficiently effective, non-toxic and cheap to find a place in routine treatment. In all these fields look out for new developments.

Sadly, we have to record the death in 1996 of our co-author Fred Miller. He made an outstanding contribution to the book. We hope the book will stand as a memorial to his remarkable work for paediatrics, and in particular for paediatric tuberculosis, in many countries. We miss him sorely.

ACKNOWLEDGEMENT OF FINANCIAL SUPPORT

Britain Nepal Medical Trust
Catholic Association for Overseas Development (CAFOD)
Chest, Heart and Stroke, Scotland
Christian Aid, United Kingdom
Community Health and Anti-tuberculosis Association of New South
.Wales, Australia
Damien Foundation, Belgium
Department of Child Health, University of Newcastle, UK
Global Tuberculosis Programme, World Health Organization
Professor Dafyd Jenkins, Wales
Landsforeningen for Hjerte-og Lungesyke, Norway
MISEREOR, Germany
NORAD, The Norwegian Agency for Development Cooperation
The Norwegian National Health Association
OXFAM, United Kingdom
Thoracic Society of Australia and New Zealand
Victoria Tuberculosis and Lung Association, Australia

In addition some translations have received support for publication
from their own national donors.

1
General Background to Clinical Tuberculosis

1: INTRODUCTION

1.1 About this book

This book is written for non-specialist hospital doctors, doctors in primary health care and other health professionals who may meet tuberculosis in the course of their work. **Almost all patients with newly diagnosed tuberculosis can be cured if properly treated**. Many will die if they are not properly treated. Therefore, as a responsible doctor or health worker

- DO NOT miss the diagnosis
- DO then give the correct treatment for the full period of time.

More than that, GOOD TREATMENT IS THE MOST IMPORTANT FORM OF PREVENTION. It makes infectious patients non-infectious. This reduces the passing on of infection in the community.

Tuberculosis is a challenging disease. Sometimes trying to make the diagnosis is like trying to solve a detective story. But if you succeed in solving the problem, you can be sure of a happy ending to the story. Modern treatment is highly successful in curing tuberculosis even in patients already infected with the HIV (AIDS) virus.

1.2 Some of the things you should know

If you are going to play your part in helping your patients, and in controlling tuberculosis in your country, you must know something about its cause. You must know where infection comes from. You must know how most people control that infection and do not get ill, but why some develop disease. The general public will also expect you to know something about the best way of **preventing tuberculosis**. If your country has a **national programme** for tuberculosis control, YOU SHOULD KNOW ABOUT IT and should play your part in making it work.

1.3   The world problem of tuberculosis

In many industrialised countries money, resources, high standards of living, and widespread chemotherapy in the last 40 years, have helped to reduce tuberculosis to a relatively minor problem. But in poorer countries it remains almost as big a problem as ever. Indeed, as their populations have increased and their tuberculosis rates have only slightly decreased, **there are probably more tuberculosis patients in the world today than there were 20 years ago.** WHO has estimated that the total number of cases in the world will rise from 7.5 million in 1990 to 10.2 million in the year 2000. Total deaths will rise from 2.5 to 3.5 million. The rise will be due partly to increases in population in developing countries and partly to the spread of the HIV virus (p 135). These rises could be stopped if many countries set up effective Tuberculosis Control Programmes (p 15).

1.4   The outlook

This may all sound depressing, but in many poor countries with high tuberculosis rates modern programmes of mass treatment efficiently applied, are showing excellent results. There are even signs that this success is beginning to make tuberculosis a little less common in some of these countries where HIV infection is low. In industrialised countries the rate of new cases (incidence rate) fell by 6–12 per cent a year after the widespread use of chemotherapy. After the introduction of good National Control Programmes WHO reports declines per year of 5 per cent for Chile, 7 per cent for Cuba, 8 per cent for Uruguay and 7 per cent for the Republic of Korea. These figures show what can be achieved. But with the explosion of HIV infection in Africa, and now in Asia, it will need very major national and international effort to achieve such results throughout the world. An increasing number of countries have made a good start. We hope you will make your own contribution in your own country.

1.5   Tuberculin surveys and annual numbers of new cases

It has been calculated that **for every 1 per cent of new annual infections** (new tuberculin positives among the population) **there will be 50–60 new smear positive cases of pulmonary tuberculosis per 100,000 population per year and an equal number of either smear-negative or non-pulmonary cases.** Using this calculation a sample tuberculin survey can be used to calculate the probable number of new cases per year in a country. (Not all experts accept the value of this method.)

1.6 Treatment

In many countries some doctors give **poor or inadequate treatment**. This is likely:

- to FAIL TO CURE the patient;
- perhaps to leave him with DRUG-RESISTANT tubercle bacilli, making it difficult for anyone else to cure him;
- to leave him alive (at least for some time) and INFECTIOUS, perhaps with drug resistant bacilli, so that he spreads the disease to others. So POOR TREATMENT is both POOR DOCTORING and POOR PUBLIC HEALTH.

Therefore, in section 2 of this chapter we give some general GUIDE-LINES and DOs and DON'Ts which will help to avoid common errors. We suggest you read these first, though we realise you yourself may not need this basic advice. Then go on (or refer when necessary) to the later parts of this book which give more detail.

2: GENERAL GUIDELINES ON THE TREATMENT OF TUBERCULOSIS

2.1 DOs and DON'Ts for doctors

2.1.1 DON'Ts. Avoid the following errors which are common in some countries:

1. Never treat a patient with probable pulmonary tuberculosis without **examining the sputum** (wherever microscopy is available). Children often have no sputum: diagnosis may have to be largely clinical (p 50).
2. Never give a **single drug alone**: drug resistance usually follows and is permanent.
3. Never **add a single drug** to a drug combination if the patient becomes worse. First make sure that he is taking the drug combination regularly. If he is, and is getting worse, his **bacilli will be resistant to all the drugs being used**. Adding one drug is the same as giving one drug alone. The patient's TB will soon be resistant to this also.
4. **Never fail to follow up the patient** and make sure he has **the full recommended course of treatment** (6 or 8 months with rifampicin-containing chemotherapy: p 167). If at all possible make sure someone sees the patient taking every dose for the first 2 months (Direct observation treatment: see p 156).
5. Never use a combination of **streptomycin and penicillin for non-tuberculous conditions**. It is seldom better than penicillin alone or

tetracyline and may induce streptomycin resistance if the patient has undiagnosed tuberculosis. Only use rifampicin to treat either tuberculosis or leprosy.

6. Never treat only on the advice of **drug firm representatives**. Their advice will be prejudiced and may well be wrong.

2.1.2 DOs.   Remember the following important and simple rules:

1. **Always examine the sputum** in a suspected case. It is the **only** certain method of diagnosis. If sputum negative, but X-ray suggestive, give antibiotics and repeat X-ray in 3 weeks: it may be transient pneumonia (or lung abscess).

2. **Only use recommended drug combinations** (p 165). It is dangerous to use drug combinations which have not been proved, or are known to be bad or risky, when virtually all patients can be cured by established methods.

3. It is very important to **convince the patient (and his family)** that **he must complete the full course of treatment** (6 or 8 months with combinations containing rifampicin and pyrazinamide) to avoid relapse. **Explanatory leaflets** are useful and should be available in your country. (Even with illiterate patients, someone in the family or village can read the leaflet.)

4. It is essential to be **kind and sympathetic** to the patient. Experience has shown that he is much more likely to come back and complete his treatment if he believes you are his friend and that you want to help him personally.

5. Remember that if a patient **has had as much as one month of treatment** in the past, and has **missed two or more consecutive months** of treatment you should give him a (different) standard **retreatment regimen** (p 167).

6. If a patient has had several courses of previous treatment (perhaps with poor drug combinations) and has now relapsed, refer him to a specialist (or obtain advice in writing). Planning treatment in such cases is difficult and a mistake can be fatal. Your National Tuberculosis Control Programme may have a special drug regimen for such patients: see p 189.

2.1.3 Cautions.   For details of recommended drug regimens see p 165. But REMEMBER:

1. **Most apparent failures** to respond to treatment, or relapse after treatment, are **because treatment has been too short**. This is due to doctor or patient not realising the importance of completing a full course with no interruptions.

   Unfortunately another reason could be that a member of staff has stolen drugs instead of giving them to the patient. Yet another reason may be that the patient has sold the drugs instead of swallowing them!

Other failures are due to bad or irregular treatment with bad drug combinations: a poorly trained doctor or health assistant may have prescribed bad treatment. Or he may have failed to instruct the patient about what pills to take, when to take them and the importance of taking them regularly. In this case the patient's TB may have developed **drug resistance** (see p 162).

2. After too short a treatment with a First Line recommended regimen such patients are likely to have tubercle bacilli **still sensitive to standard drugs**. They can safely be put back on a **First Line regimen**.
3. If you consider you must give rifampicin (and if it is not yet included in your national programme):
   a) Make sure the patient can afford **the full course of treatment**. If treatment is too short he will relapse.
   b) Give **one of the recommended drug regimens** (p 165). Other regimens may result in failure, the development of **resistant tubercle bacilli** or **early relapse**.

2.2 Guidelines on tuberculosis for non-medical health staff

As a doctor you should ensure that all your staff know and act upon the following summary.

> Tuberculosis can be cured
> THE PATIENT'S LIFE DEPENDS ON YOU

2.2.1 Tuberculosis is an **infectious disease** spread through cough and sputum. Therefore DO ALL YOU CAN TO DISCOURAGE SPITTING. Never spit yourself. When coughing cover your mouth with your hands.

2.2.2 Symptoms of tuberculosis If a patient has any of the following, consider him a 'Tuberculosis Suspect' (see p 90):

- cough for more than 3 weeks
- coughing blood
- pain in the chest for more than 3 weeks
- fever for more than 3 weeks

All these can be due to other diseases but **sputum must be tested** if any are present.

2.2.3 Sputum examination is much more reliable than X-ray. If 3 sputa **negative** give simple treatment (not tuberculosis drugs) but repeat sputum examination if symptoms continue and/or refer to a tuberculosis clinic or a doctor. Diagnosis in children can be difficult (p. 44). If possible refer to a doctor.

2.2.4   If **sputum is positive** tuberculosis can be easily cured if the patient takes his full treatment (p 154).

2.2.5   Symptoms soon clear but **treatment must continue regularly for the full period** recommended (see p 156). Otherwise tuberculosis comes back and the period of treatment has to start all over again.

2.2.6   BCG is a good protection against tuberculosis in children, especially against the fatal forms of tuberculous meningitis and miliary tuberculosis.

DOs and DON'Ts in tuberculosis

- DO always **examine the sputum** when there are symptoms suggestive of possible tuberculosis.
- DO make sure the patient understands that he needs a **full period of treatment though symptoms will soon clear**. (Give the patient a leaflet on treatment if available.)
- DO explain this to his relatives.
- DO be **kind and sympathetic:** then the patient is more likely to come back for drug supplies and continue treatment. Think of him as a friend you want to help.
- DO examine all **family/home contacts**, especially if they are ill.
- DO put his name in the **tuberculosis register** and give him a **treatment card** with the next date of attendance. Make sure he understands and remembers the date.
- DO send someone to his home if he **fails to come back** on the date. (A letter is usually less effective but may be all you can do.)
- DO check frequently your **supplies of anti-tuberculosis drugs** and see that you don't run out.
- DON'T forget that **any chronic cougher may have tuberculosis**, especially if he or she has fever and loss of weight.
- DON'T forget to **test the sputum**.
- DON'T forget to **follow up patients who fail to come back** and persuade them to complete treatment.

AGAIN
TUBERCULOSIS CAN BE CURED
YOU CAN DO MORE THAN ANYONE ELSE
TO SAVE THE PATIENT'S LIFE

3: THE BATTLE BETWEEN THE TUBERCLE BACILLI AND THE PATIENT

3.1   Causes of tuberculosis: the bacillus

OVERWHELMING IMPORTANCE	Minor importance
TUBERCLE BACILLUS (*Mycobacterium tuberculosis*)	West Africa (*Mycobacterium africanum*)
Rare and of slight importance (See text)	
Bovine tubercle bacillus (*Mycobacterium bovis*)	Non-tuberculous mycobacteria

Figure 1   *Causes of tuberculosis and related diseases* in high prevalence countries

3.1.1   Though there are some other sorts of bacilli the tubercle bacillus (*Mycobacterium tuberculosis*: TB) is the **main cause of tuberculosis all over the world**.

3.1.2   A slightly different type of TB, *Mycobacterium africanum*, occurs in Africa. The only important difference is that it is often resistant to thioacetazone (Tb1) (p 184).

3.1.3   The **bovine tubercle bacillus** (*Mycobacterium bovis*) at one time caused much infection in cattle in Europe and the Americas. Infection was often passed on to man through milk. With control of cattle tuberculosis by killing of infected animals and pasteurisation of milk, these countries have largely prevented bovine tuberculosis in man. Disease can occur in cattle, camels and dromedaries in low income countries. It is thought to be rare but we do not yet have enough information on this. Human infection from bovine bacilli seems not to occur in India. Elsewhere in Asia it is thought to be rare, perhaps because in many countries milk is boiled before use. In others it is not used at all. We still need more information about how much bovine tuberculosis exists in Africa and Asia, both in animals and man.

3.1.4   **Non-tuberculous mycobacteria** include a wide range of bacterial species. Many are harmless. They are common in the environments of many high prevalence countries but they seldom cause disease. However, harmless infection in humans can give rise to a weakly positive tuberculin skin test. (Disease from these bacilli has become relatively more important in some developed countries, such as parts of USA and Australia, where ordinary tuberculosis has now greatly decreased. It may also develop in patients infected with HIV. As these bacilli are resistant to most commonly used drugs the disease is more difficult to treat (p 199).)

Nearly all tuberculosis in high prevalence countries is caused by the common tubercle bacillus, *M. tuberculosis* (TB), so that is what most of this book is about.

3.2   Infection and disease

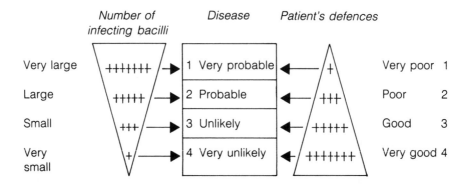

Figure 2   *Probability of developing tuberculous disease.* The influence of the numbers of infecting bacilli and the strength of the patient's defences

3.2.1   In the past, when tuberculosis was widespread in industrialised countries it was possible to show by skin-testing with **tuberculin** (p 200) that most young adults had become infected. But only a small proportion (about 10 per cent) developed the disease. This is still what happens in most high prevalence countries.

3.2.2   Whether **infection goes on to disease** (Figure 2) depends on:

- the *size of the infecting dose*, i.e. how many TB are inhaled;
- the *defences* of the person infected (host resistance).

3.2.3   In some cases infection may rapidly go on to disease. In others TB may **remain 'dormant'**, with a few 'sleeping' bacilli kept under control by the defences. But some later lowering of the patient's defences, e.g. by malnutrition, by another disease (such as HIV infection) or just old age,

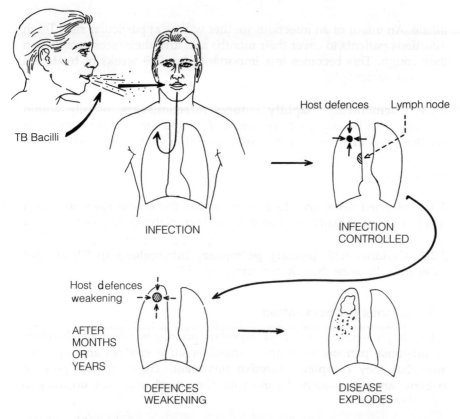

Figure 3 *TB infection and host's (patient's) defences.* At first the patient's defences may keep the TB under control. After months or years his/her defences may weaken, e.g. from malnutrition or another disease. Then the disease starts to spread in the lung. A cavity may develop in the lung. The sputum may become positive for TB and the patient infect children or other people

may allow the dormant TB to multiply and cause disease (Figure 3). In most people their host defences either kill off all the bacilli or, perhaps more often, keep them suppressed and under long-term control.

3.3 Where infection comes from (sources of infection)

3.3.1 Human SPUTUM is far the most important source. Coughing, talking and spitting produce very small droplets containing TB which float in the air. These may be inhaled and cause disease.

3.3.2 Patients with sputum positive on **direct smear** (i.e. TB visible under the microscope) are much more infectious, because they are producing far more TB, than those only positive on culture. The closer someone lives to the patient, the bigger the dose of TB he will probably inhale. An infant of an infectious mother will be at particular risk. Teach infectious patients to cover their mouths and turn their faces away when they cough. This becomes less important after 2–3 weeks of treatment (see next paragraph).

3.3.3 Chemotherapy rapidly reduces infectiousness, usually within 2 weeks. This is why **good treatment** of all sputum positive patients **is far the most effective method of prevention**. But if treatment is not continued for the full period the patient may **relapse** and again become infectious.

3.3.4 Infected urine and discharges etc. are theoretical risks but much less important, usually because they contain relatively few bacilli.

3.3.5 Children with **primary pulmonary tuberculosis** (p 50) **are not infectious**, because they do not cough out TB.

3.4   Lessons for prevention

3.4.1 In prevention, your most important priority as a doctor is therefore to **diagnose** patients with direct smear positive sputum and to make sure that they **complete effective treatment**. These sputum positive patients are also usually the most ill. They need treatment urgently to save their lives.

3.4.2 Sterilisation of sputum, bedclothes, etc.

a) Direct **sunlight** kills TB in 5 minutes. Exposure to sunlight is therefore a convenient method in the tropics. (But bacilli may survive for years in the dark: much spread of infection probably occurs in dark houses or huts.)

b) **Sodium hypochlorite** (1 per cent) liquifies sputum and kills TB rapidly but has to be used in glass jars as it damages metal. It also bleaches dyed material if dropped on it. Add to the sputum twice its volume of hypochlorite. (TB may resist 5 per cent phenol for several hours.)

c) **Heat**: TB are destroyed in 20 minutes at 60°C and in 5 minutes at 70°C.

d) **Paper handkerchiefs** should be burnt as soon as possible after use. (Old newspapers or other similar material can also be used and then burnt.)

e) Exposure to **air and sunlight** is a good and simple method, particularly in the tropics, for dealing with blankets, woollens, cottons etc.

3.4.3 Environmental hygiene. The aim is to reduce the risk from the sputum of undiagnosed infectious patients. There is a limit to what can be achieved in poorer countries but the following could help:

a) *Reduce overcrowding* wherever possible (which also reduces other infectious respiratory diseases, such as pneumonia in infants).
b) Improve *ventilation* of houses.
c) Help everyone to think *spitting* a nasty and unacceptable habit. (In countries where tobacco and betel nut chewing is common, health education to stop this cancer-producing habit will also reduce spitting.) Teach that spitting spreads disease.

3.5 How a person resists infection (host defences)

Many things affect the way our bodies fight the tubercle bacillus. These include:

3.5.1 Age and sex (Table 1, p 12). There is little difference between boys and girls up to puberty. Infants and young children of both sexes have weak defences. Up to age 2 infection is particularly liable to result in the most fatal forms, **miliary tuberculosis** and **tuberculous meningitis**, due to bloodstream spread. After age one, and before puberty, an infected child may develop miliary or meningitis, or one of the more chronic disseminated types of tuberculosis, particularly **lymph node, bone** or **joint disease**. Before puberty the lung part of the **primary lesion** (p 30) usually just affects that local area, though cavities like those in adults may be seen in Africa or Asia in children with severe malnutrition, especially girls aged 10–14. The lymph node part of the primary complex may also give rise to lung collapse etc. (p 33). In Europe and North America, when tuberculosis was common, the **peak incidence of pulmonary tuberculosis** was usually in young adults. The male rate continued fairly high at all ages but the female rate tended to drop rapidly after the childbearing years. Women often developed pulmonary tuberculosis following childbirth. Limited information from Africa and India seems to indicate a somewhat different pattern. The prevalence of pulmonary tuberculosis seems to increase with age in both sexes. In women the overall prevalence is lower and the rise with age less steep than in men. In women it reaches a maximum at age 40–50 and then falls. In men it goes on rising at least to age 60.

3.5.2 Nutrition. There is very good evidence that **starvation** or **malnutrition** reduces resistance to the disease. This is a very important factor in poorer communities, both in adults and children.

3.5.3 Toxic factors. **Tobacco smoking** and high **alcohol** intake are important in reducing body defences. So are **corticosteroid drugs** and other **immunosuppressants** used for treating certain diseases.

Table 1   *Factors affecting the patient's defences against tuberculosis.* Age and sex. *If infection occurs at a particular age (lefthand column) the number of +s in the righthand column shows how probable it is that the patient will develop that particular form of tuberculosis.* Other factors: *The number of +s in the righthand column shows the importance of that particular factor in damaging the patient's power to resist the bacilli.*

Age and sex	Patient liable to develop
Under 1 year	Miliary tuberculosis++ Tuberculous meningitis++
Age 1 to puberty	Primary lung lesion+ Chronic disseminated tuberculosis, e.g. bone and joint+ miliary tuberculosis+ tuberculous meningitis+
Adolescent/young adult	PULMONARY TUBERCULOSIS+++

Middle age
  Males
  Females
	
	PULMONARY TUBERCULOSIS++
	PULMONARY TUBERCULOSIS+

Old age
  Males
  Females
	
	PULMONARY TUBERCULOSIS++
	PULMONARY TUBERCULOSIS+−

Other factors	
Factor	Importance
MALNUTRITION	+++
TOXIC:	
Tobacco	+
Alcohol	+
Corticosteroids	+
Immunosuppressants	+
OTHER DISEASES:	
HIV infection	+++
Diabetes	+
Leprosy	+
Silicosis	+
Leukaemia	+
Measles } in a Whooping cough } child	+++
Poor environment	? +
Race	? +
IMMUNOLOGICAL	
AIDS	+++
Alcohol	+
Tobacco	+
Other toxic	+

3.5.4 The importance of risk factors. In Table 1 the important risk factors which may increase your country's **incidence of tuberculosis** are age, HIV/AIDS and the 'poverty complex' (see 3.5.5 below). In the poverty complex, malnutrition and overcrowding are probably the most important. But as a doctor remember that if you see a patient with one of the risk factors, always remember the possibility of tuberculosis.

3.5.5 Poverty. This leads to bad and overcrowded housing or poor work conditions. These may lower defences as well as making infection more likely. People living in such conditions are often also badly nourished. The whole complex of poverty makes it easier for the TB to cause disease.

3.5.6 Race. It is difficult to separate the possible effects of race from other factors, such as poverty. However there is good evidence that isolated populations, for instance Innuits (Eskimos) or Native Americans, when they met the disease for the first time had poor defences. Tuberculosis spread very rapidly and caused a high mortality. In Europe or China, where tuberculosis had been common for many centuries, those with congenitally poor defences had probably died early, often before they had children. The survivors probably had more 'natural' resistance to the disease. But in populations where the disease was new affected people often died in a few months from so-called 'galloping consumption'.

3.6 Lessons for prevention

3.6.1 Many of the factors we have been describing can be removed only by economic or government action to decrease poverty and improve nutrition. In industrialised countries this has been perhaps the most important factor in the long-term decrease of tuberculosis over the last century. As a doctor, you may not be able to do much about this. But in recent years LARGE SCALE EFFECTIVE TREATMENT has speeded up the decrease by reducing the numbers of infectious people in the population. You can and must contribute to this in your own area. The first priority is to make sure that all sputum positive patients complete effective treatment.

3.6.2 **Reducing national tobacco consumption** will help to prevent tuberculosis, as well as preventing lung (and other) cancers, coronary heart disease, chronic bronchitis etc. As a doctor, and a leader of opinion, you can do a lot about this. In particular, **do not smoke yourself** and NEVER in front of patients.

3.6.3   **Reduction in national alcohol consumption** will also help. YOU SHOULD THEREFORE SUPPORT NATIONAL NO SMOKING AND ALCOHOL REDUCTION CAMPAIGNS, which will prevent other important diseases besides tuberculosis.

3.7   BCG

3.7.1   BCG is a vaccine consisting of live bacilli which have lost their virulence. (The bacilli originally came from a strain of bovine TB grown for many years in the laboratory.) BCG stimulates immunity, increasing the body's defences without itself causing damage. Following BCG vaccination TB may enter the body but in most cases the body's increased defences will control or kill them.

3.7.2   Controlled trials in several Western countries, where most children are well-nourished, have shown that BCG **can give 80 per cent protection** against tuberculosis for as long as 15 years if administered **before** first infection (i.e. to tuberculin negative children).

3.7.3   However, large scale trials of the same type in USA and India have failed to show benefit. But a number of smaller scale trials in **infants** in poor countries have shown important protection, especially against miliary tuberculosis and tuberculous meningitis.

3.7.4   The present recommendation by WHO and the International Union Against Tuberculosis and Lung Disease is that in countries with high tuberculosis prevalence BCG SHOULD BE GIVEN AS A ROUTINE TO ALL INFANTS (but with a few exceptions, such as active AIDS). The normal dose is 0.05 ml in neonates and infants and 0.1 ml in older children and adults.

3.7.5   The **effect of BCG probably lasts about 15 years**, at least in a well-nourished population. Some countries therefore try to repeat BCG about the age of 15 (e.g. in school-leavers). But it is difficult to cover the whole population at this age. And its value when given at this age in tropical countries has not yet been scientifically proved.

3.7.6   Because the main effect of infant vaccination is to protect children, and because children with primary tuberculosis are not usually infectious, BCG has little effect in reducing the number of adult infectious cases in the population. To reduce these, IT IS MUCH MORE IMPORTANT TO GIVE GOOD TREATMENT TO ALL SPUTUM POSITIVE PATIENTS. But of course we should give BCG as a routine to all infants as a protection in childhood (See 3.7.4 above).

3.7.7   In a number of countries health care workers are tuberculin tested before starting work that may expose them to possible infection with TB. If negative they are given BCG. This is particularly important if they may be exposed to multidrug resistant TB. It is also very important for workers in bacteriological and pathology departments.

4: TUBERCULOSIS CONTROL PROGRAMMES

Table 2   *Essentials of tuberculosis control programmes*

---

1. *National and local agreement* to programme (para 4.1.3)
2. National and local *health education* about TB (para 4.1.5)
3. *Case-finding* by routine sputum microscopy for TB in those with symptoms (para 4.2.2–3)
4. *Standard supervised treatment* (para 4.2.5–6)
5. Methods for *recalling defaulters* (para 4.2.6)
6. *Standard records* (para 4.2.7) and monitoring
7. Ensuring uninterrupted drug and other *supplies* (para 4.2.8)
8. Regular *training* and *retraining* (para 4.2.9)
9. *BCG vaccination* for the newborn (para 4.2.10)
10. Examination of *family contacts* (para 4.2.11)

Note: Most of the above, especially items 1–8, are essential components of WHO 'DOTS' programme (Directly Observed Treatment Shortcourse: see also p 156).

4.1   Introduction

4.1.1   More and more high prevalence countries now have control programmes for tuberculosis, which have been nationally agreed (Table 2). In a number of countries the programme is combined with the Leprosy Control Programme. It is important that you should play your part in the national control programme if there is one in your country. It is poor doctoring to be ignorant of the programme and even worse to know about it and not to do your best to follow it out in your own work.

With the increase in HIV infection in some countries national programmes will have to take account of this in both diagnosis and treatment (See p 135).

4.1.2   The aim of a national programme is to use limited resources to prevent, diagnose and treat the disease in the best and most economical way.

4.1.3   Experience has shown that the programme is most likely to succeed if it has been fully **discussed by representatives of all those who will take part in it**. This includes central, intermediate (regional, provincial) and district administrators; specialist and general doctors, nurses and health workers from institutes, laboratories, hospitals and primary care; representatives of both health and finance ministries; and representatives, politicians and others, of the general population and local communities.

4.1.4 After central agreement of all these, it is important to hold seminars in different parts of the country at local levels. It is most important that representatives of the **local population** are consulted so that arrangements can fit in with local customs and convenience. For instance diagnostic and treatment sessions should take place when country people are likely to be in town for the local market day and at times when patients can get away from their work. Health workers must find out the **local beliefs about tuberculosis,** so that education about the disease and its treatment can be adapted to those beliefs.

4.1.5 The seminars should be followed by national and local **health education campaigns** (television, radio, newspapers, schools) about tuberculosis. They must also tell people about the programme, so that they know how tuberculosis can be diagnosed and treated, so that they know it can always be cured if proper treatment is taken and so that they have some idea how it is spread and how it can be prevented.

4.1.6 *Note on local beliefs.* Local beliefs about tuberculosis and its cause will obviously vary in different countries, different areas, different cultures and even different groups of the population in the same area. Religion, caste, tribe or degree of education may influence people's ideas. In some places people believe that tuberculosis is due to evil spirits which have got into the patient. Even where people know that tuberculosis is an infectious disease, they may think a particular person has got the disease because he has been bewitched. In one area most ordinary people thought that a patient usually caught tuberculosis from the stick which was used for cleaning the teeth. In another people thought that the symptoms were often due to a sin, such as adultery.

You may be able to persuade local healers to send patients with possible tuberculosis to health centres for diagnosis and treatment. Explain to them that if they try to treat these patients themselves they will fail. This will be bad for their local reputation and their practice.

In many cultures people think that tuberculosis is hereditary. This idea is not surprising. Tuberculosis is an infectious disease. Often several members of the family, sometimes in different generations, may develop it. Unfortunately this idea often means that people are ashamed of the disease. They feel that it is a disgrace to the family. If a daughter gets tuberculosis the family may be afraid that they will never find her a husband. This idea may remain even after she is obviously cured. If it is a common idea in the community in which you work, try to educate opinion leaders so that patients and their families do not suffer from this additional anxiety. In our experience the idea disappears when the community realises that good treatment is easily available and almost always cures the disease. Cured patients may be able to help in educating both new patients and the community.

4.1.7 If your country has a **National Programme make sure that you and your staff know its details and help to make it successful**.

4.2 Components of a national tuberculosis control programme (Table 2, p 15)

4.2.1 Details of model national programmes are given in:
Tuberculosis Guide for Low Income Countries. 4th edn. Enarson, D.A., Rieder, H.L., Arnadottir, T., Trébucq, A. Paris: International Union Against Tuberculosis and Lung Disease, 1996.
(See Reference list p 215).

We only give a brief outline here:

4.2.2 Casefinding

a)   Examine the sputum for TB of all patients who have had a **cough and sputum for more than 3 weeks**. (Cough due to an acute infection will usually be clearing up, or will have gone, by 3 weeks. Cough due to tuberculosis will be unchanged or getting worse.) This is particularly important if the patient also has **loss of weight, fever, pain in the chest** or has **coughed up blood** (Figure 4). Some patients have these last symptoms without any chronic cough. (See also p 90.)
      If a patient has any of these symptoms think of him as a 'tuberculosis suspect'.

b)   Investigate and follow up any patient with an X-ray of chest showing a shadow which could be due to tuberculosis. In particular, examine his sputum for TB. But indiscriminate mass X-ray of the population is expensive and unreliable. We do **not** recommend it. Sputum testing is much more reliable. (See 4.2.3 c)).

c)   **'Active' and 'passive' casefinding**. Most patients with tuberculosis who are ill and with a positive sputum will attend some health facility (health centre, hospital, out-patient clinic or private doctor),

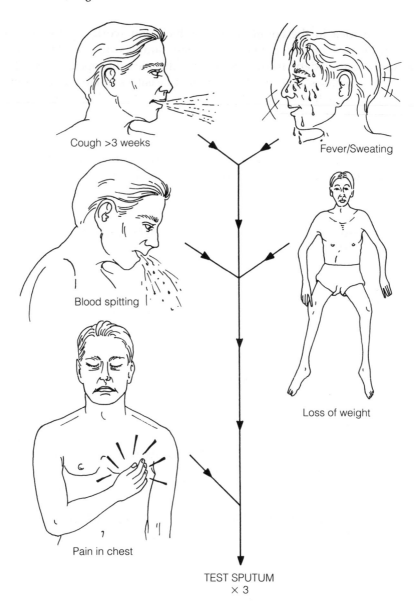

Cough >3 weeks

Fever/Sweating

Blood spitting

Loss of weight

Pain in chest

TEST SPUTUM
× 3

Figure 4   *Diagnosing lung tuberculosis*. The most important symptoms

but **will be diagnosed only if their sputum is routinely examined for TB**. This is 'passive casefinding'. 'Active casefinding' is going to people's homes and asking them to produce sputum for testing. This is very expensive and gives much fewer positives. 'Passive casefinding' is much more economical, provided it is properly done: it is the standard method in the vast majority of national programmes. If people in a community know that in their area patients with tuberculosis get good treatment from understanding and friendly health workers, and are cured, then far more people come looking for help. Once patients who come with symptoms are properly tested, properly treated and are properly cured, then it may be time to go on to active casefinding and search for the less urgent cases, e.g. those positive on culture only.

4.2.3 Diagnosis

a) **Microscopy of the sputum is far, far the most reliable** (and the cheapest) **method** which you can use in most places. Try to have three specimens examined. If only one is positive and the others negative, it is best to confirm with a further positive (because errors, clerical or other, can occur).

b) Because chronic cough may be due to smoking, chronic bronchitis, etc., many specimens of sputum will be negative. In good programmes only 5–10 per cent of patients usually turn out to have a positive sputum. Where there is little 'smoker's cough' the figure may be 15–20 per cent. You must test all patients with chronic cough, especially those with weight loss or other symptoms which might be due to tuberculosis. Do this wherever you work: in primary care, clinic, hospital or private practice. Not to do this is bad medicine.

c) **X-ray chest** (see p 95). Tuberculosis is difficult to diagnose with certainty on an X-ray alone. **Never treat such a patient without having examined the sputum**. X-rays are expensive and unreliable. Patients are often treated for tuberculosis when they do not have it. X-rays are sometimes needed for difficult individual problems, in particular for HIV-positive tuberculosis suspects, but are not suitable for mass case-finding in high prevalence countries.

d) **Tuberculin test** (see p 200) is often a less reliable method for diagnosis in poorer countries. Owing to malnutrition, other disease such as HIV infection, or the severity of tuberculosis it can be weak or negative even when the patient (adult or child) has active tuberculous disease. So that a negative tuberculin test does not exclude tuberculosis. But a **strongly positive test in a child suspected of tuberculosis can be very helpful**. Remember a child can have a weakly positive test due to BCG and that in many countries a high proportion of adults will have a positive test due to childhood infection.

4.2.4 Laboratory services

a) **Microscopy** must be made widely available, as near the patient as possible. This is far the most important means of diagnosis. But it must be well supervised and reliable. At first this may only be possible at District level. See Reference 11 p 215.

b) **Culture** for TB may later be made available as services develop. Only use it for patients with X-ray shadows suspicious of tuberculosis. Culture makes a definite diagnosis possible in milder cases which are negative on microscopy.

c) Testing for **drug resistance** is too expensive for routine use. It is desirable to have a national reference laboratory which can monitor drug resistance trends in a sample of patients, so that the authorities can modify standard treatment methods if necessary. Reliable resistance tests for isoniazid, rifampicin and streptomycin can be useful in planning retreatment in a difficult case, but in many countries will not be available for this purpose (see p 192).

4.2.5 Treatment.   The national programme will state:

a) **Standard treatment for new cases** of sputum positive pulmonary tuberculosis and severe forms of non-pulmonary tuberculosis. Both WHO and IUATLD now recommend short-course chemotherapy containing rifampicin at least in the intensive phase. These regimens last 6–8 months: see p 167 for details. Some poorer countries still use a 12-month regimen not using the more expensive rifampicin and pyrazinamide. Or they may use this regimen only for sputum negative pulmonary tuberculosis.

b) Patients who **relapse**, who return after **default**, or who appear to have **failed to respond** to standard treatment. WHO and IUATLD now recommend one of the **retreatment regimens** outlined on p 167. This will be effective in most such patients. Failure in most is due to not having taken full treatment, not to drug resistance. The retreatment regimen will be effective when there is resistance only to one or two drugs. In fact 'chronic cases' who have had repeated bad treatment may not respond because of multiple resistance: see p 192 for discussion of the problem.

c) **New smear negative pulmonary tuberculosis and milder cases of extrapulmonary**. Many programmes (and WHO) recommend less intensive regimens: see p 167. Some programmes think it less confusing to give the same regimen to all newly diagnosed patients.

4.2.6 Treatment supervision.   This should be laid down in the programme. The whole success of the programme depends on good supervision of treatment. Ideally treatment should be directly observed (that is the patient is seen to take each dose), at least for the first two important months. In some programmes the patient is admitted to hospital for the first 2 months. In others he is admitted to a hostel near a clinic. In yet others he attends a clinic or health post for each dose: if this is the method, make sure he is not kept waiting. If he is kept waiting he may not come back. In some rural areas directly observed treatment may have to be done by some local responsible person or volunteer. The patient gets to know the person. That bond decreases default. The programme will lay down a method for recalling patients who have failed to report for treatment or failed to collect their drugs. If no such system exists in your area it is important to make your own arrangements (see p 158).

4.2.7 Records

a) In order to run a successful Tuberculosis Control Programme there must be good records.

> • Records are important for you in your **Clinic/Health Centre** so that you can make sure that you fully follow up your patients and that all patients complete treatment.
> • Returns from Clinics/Health Centres are important at *District/Area* level so that administrators can make sure you have the drugs and materials to diagnose and treat your patients. They can also compare the work of different clinics and compare their own results with those of other Districts.
> • Returns from Districts are important at *National* level for evaluating patient progress, comparing Districts and planning supplies.

> Filling up forms is a nuisance but it is an essential part of a good National Tuberculosis Control Programme. Make sure you and your staff do it carefully and well. It is important not only for your own day-to-day work. It is also an important step to your getting the materials and support you need for your patients.
> The programme will state the methods for recording numbers of sputum tested, numbers found positive, routine follow-up of patients with regular sputum tests to ensure sputum-conversion to negative, deaths, defaults, relapses and numbers successfully completing treatment. The easiest way to collect relevant information on casefinding and evaluation of treatment is to have a 'District Tuberculosis Register' in every District (area). This should contain each patient's name, address, site of disease, whether sputum positive on diagnosis, and results of smear examinations at follow-up until treatment is completed.
> This record will give an indication of how enthusiastically health workers are looking for patients and how successful they are in curing them with a full course of treatment.

b) The programme may define the type of patient to be recorded, e.g.:
New patients:

- Sputum positive pulmonary tuberculosis: at least two direct smear positive sputa.
- Culture positive pulmonary tuberculosis: in areas where culture is possible.
- Sputum negative pulmonary tuberculosis: diagnosis made on clinical and/or X-ray: if possible this diagnosis should only be made by a doctor.
- Non-pulmonary tuberculosis: Confirmed by bacteriology or histology. Clinical diagnosis, usually by a doctor: diagnosis will include organ affected, e.g. miliary tuberculosis, tuberculous meningitis, spinal tuberculosis.

Relapse/retreatment patients: Patients who have been previously diagnosed as tuberculous, who have had treatment (complete or partial) with improvement or disappearance of symptoms for one or more months. He/she has now returned with clinical and/or bacteriological (e.g. positive sputum) evidence of active tuberculosis.
Treatment failures: defined by WHO as a new patient who is still sputum smear positive 5 months or more after starting standard treatment. (This is most often due to failure to make sure he has taken his full course of treatment. It is much less often due to drug resistance.)
Patients lost to observation (defaulters): Patients who have failed to attend for 2 or more months in spite of every effort to trace them: the exact definition may vary in different programmes.
Transfers out: Patients who have moved to another area. Only include such a patient if you have made arrangements for his/her treatment at a health facility in the new area.

c) **Record forms and registers.** Your national programme will provide these. For examples see References 1 and 2, p 215.
d) All this will build up a picture of national progress in casefinding and treatment. It will also show up local differences, which may be due either to differences in the amount of tuberculosis or differences in the enthusiasm of the health workers. Make sure you are one of the enthusiasts who do a good job.

4.2.8 Regular and uninterrupted supplies of drugs and materials for microscopy (4.2.4 above) are essential to success.

4.2.9 Repeated central and local **training sessions and seminars** will compare success rates in diagnosing and treating patients in different places and help health workers to learn from one another.

4.2.10 BCG vaccination should be given to all newborn children (with certain exceptions: see p 14) through the national Expanded Programme of Immunisation. All infants should be vaccinated within a year of birth.

4.2.11 FAMILY CONTACTS of tuberculous patients.

a) A patient with a positive sputum will often infect members of his or her own family, especially children. Obviously this is because a family lives in close contact. If your patient has a positive sputum examine his family to find **who he may have infected**.

b) On the other hand, if the patient you first diagnose is a child with tuberculosis, examine the family to see **who may have infected the child**. It might be a parent or a grandparent. Of course you will also look for anyone else in the family who has been infected.

How to manage family contacts

1. **Figure 5** is a flow chart on how to manage a **child contact** if you **can** do a tuberculin test (see p 200).
   Remember the tuberculin test *may be negative*:

   - if the child has been infected with TB only recently and has not yet become tuberculin positive;
   - if the child is malnourished or ill with another disease (see p 46);
   - if the child is very ill with tuberculosis.

   Remember that it is particularly important to give preventive ('prophylactic') isoniazid treatment, as in Figure 5, to children aged 5 years or less. These young children are in particular danger from the severe forms of tuberculosis, miliary or meningitis.

2. **Figure 6** is a flow chart on how to manage a **child contact** if you **cannot** do a tuberculin test.

3. **Figure 7** is a flow chart on how to manage an **adult contact**. Here a tuberculin test is less useful, as many adults will be tuberculin positive.

   Remember that it is important to examine **all** adults living in the family home. In particular remember the grandparents. One of them may be the infector.

---

c) Remember that a recently infected child (or adult) may still have a negative tuberculin test and appear well. A positive test, and perhaps illness, may only show later.

d) Your national tuberculosis control programme may state a routine for managing family contacts. If so, follow it.

   If you have no national programme, or it does not provide a routine plan, we suggest you follow the guidance and flow charts which follow. How you manage contacts will depend partly on whether you can do **tuberculin tests** and whether you can do X-rays.

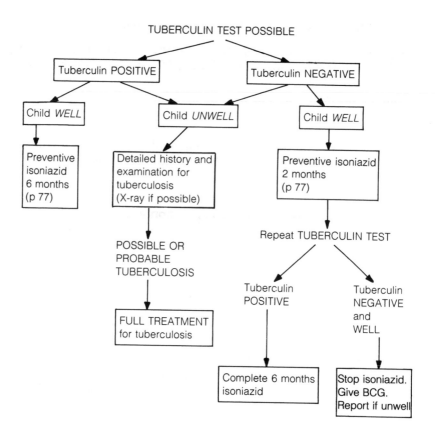

Figure 5   Flow chart: *how to manage a child contact* of a newly diagnosed patient with tuberculosis

4.3   Conclusions

If your country has a national Tuberculosis Control Programme, make sure you are familiar with it. In particular:

- **Make sure that you test the sputum of any patient who could possibly have tuberculosis.**
- Give **treatment** in accordance with the national programme. DON'T TAKE SHORT CUTS OR USE SOME NEW UNTRIED CHEMO-THERAPY. EITHER MAY BE FATAL FOR YOUR PATIENT.

4.4   Integration of control programme into primary health care

4.4.1   Many National Tuberculosis Programmes were started as programmes exclusively devoted to tuberculosis. Few of these managed to

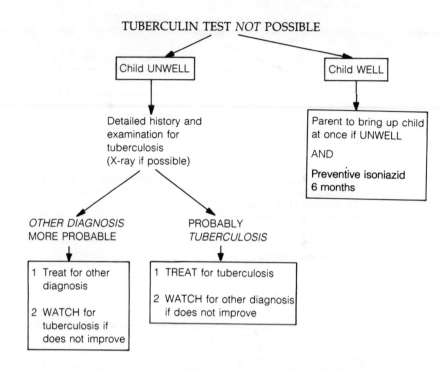

Figure 6 Flow chart: *how to manage a child contact* of a newly diagnosed patient with tuberculosis

cover the whole population. As a result WHO now recommends that all health programmes in developing countries, including those for tuberculosis, should be carried out through the routine services. Tuberculosis experts will help to plan, supervise, train and retrain. When the programme is fully established the primary care workers will decide about testing sputum for TB. If the sputum is positive the primary care worker will start routine treatment. He or she will refer difficult cases for expert advice.

4.4.2 In any programme, the resources given to tuberculosis must depend on how important a health problem it is in that country or area.

4.4.3 Although it is easy to accept this idea in theory, making it really work, or switching over from a previous 'specialised' programme to a programme working well through routine services is **very difficult in practice**: the aims must be to rouse the enthusiasm of primary care workers; to praise their successes; to help them overcome their failures;

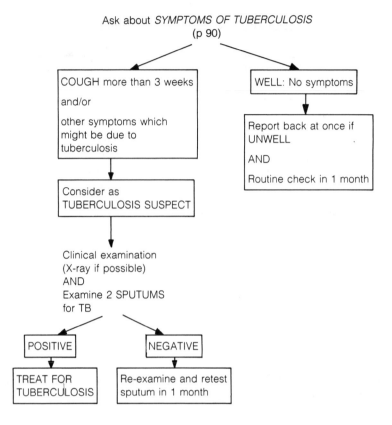

Figure 7 Flow chart: *how to manage an adult contact* of a recently diagnosed patient with tuberculosis

to **train, train and retrain** – not only in techniques but, above all, in **management**; to get workers regularly together to discuss their problems; and above all to provide **leadership** to which workers so readily respond. All these can help in achieving success. It may be best to get diagnosis and treatment first working well at Provincial and District level. Then it should be possible to move at least some diagnosis and treatment out to Health Posts/Health Centres etc.

Make sure that you yourself make your own contribution to leadership, to developing the programme and to making sure it goes on working.

4.4.4 In defeating tuberculosis **management skills** are every bit as important as clinical skills. There must be a **strong team of experts with the authority** and enthusiasm to ensure that the programme is carried out at primary care level. The team should also be available to give expert advice when needed.

4.4.5 After all, **tuberculosis** can virtually **always be cured, and spread of tuberculosis can be prevented**. We have the tools to do the job. This book is to help you to use some of these tools more effectively.

2
Tuberculosis in Children

When you use this chapter in your work in a health centre or district hospital you will be looking for answers to some or all of the following questions.

1. What happens when a child is first infected with tuberculosis?
2. Is the child I have just seen likely to have tuberculosis?
3. How does tuberculosis show itself in children?
4. How must I help the child I think has tuberculosis?

All these questions are linked together. To answer one or all of them you need to know how children are infected and the changes which follow a first infection at different ages.

The chapter is therefore set out in five sections. Together these will help you to answer the questions you ask yourself and meet your difficulties.

1. Infection with tuberculosis (p 29)
2. Meeting the child who might have tuberculosis (p 44)
3. How tuberculosis shows in children (p 50)
4. How you can help and treat tuberculous children (p 76)
5. HIV infection, AIDS (Acquired ImmunoDeficiency Syndrome) and tuberculosis in children (p 82)

1: INFECTION WITH TUBERCULOSIS

1.1 How children are infected

1.1.1 From coughing adults. When an adult coughs many small drops of liquid (spit) are forced into the air. If that adult has tuberculosis in his or her lungs many of the drops carry bacilli.

The largest of the drops fall to the ground. But the smallest, which cannot be seen, remain in the air and move with it.

Out of doors or in well ventilated rooms the small drops are carried away in the moving air. But in closed rooms, huts or small spaces they remain in the air and increase in number as the person continues to cough. Everyone sharing the room with the 'cougher' and breathing the same air runs the risk of breathing in tubercle bacilli (TB). Those nearest to the person coughing are most likely to do so.

The danger is greatest when the 'cougher' does not take any care. He should cover his or her mouth, turn away from the other persons or children and spit into something which is then covered and kept closed.

So the infectious mother is a danger to her infant or children. Both parents are dangerous in small living or sleeping spaces. So would be an infectious teacher in the classroom, an infectious doctor or dentist in the clinic or health centre or an infectious nurse or midwife or health worker in the home or hospital, a shopkeeper in his shop or a bus driver in his bus.

Almost always when **young children** are infected the **infection comes from a member of the family group or a near neighbour**. When **older children** are infected and the immediate family is clear, look for a possible infector in school, in clinic, in church, in public transport or wherever children come in contact with adults inside buildings or small spaces.

In these situations, the bacilli are taken into the lungs with the breath and this is much the commonest way of infection.

But it is not the only way.

1.1.2 From food or milk. TB can reach children in milk or food and infection can then begin in the mouth or intestine. Milk can carry bovine TB if cows in the area have tuberculosis and the milk is not boiled before use. When that happens the primary infection is in the intestine, or sometimes in the tonsils. But, as mentioned on p 7, human infection with bovine bacilli seems to be uncommon in many high prevalence countries.

1.1.3 Through the skin. Unbroken skin seems to resist TB if they fall upon its surface. But if there has been a recent cut or break TB may get in and cause an infection as they do in the lungs. As might be expected, skin infection is most likely on exposed surfaces such as the face or legs or feet or less often on the arm or hand. These primary lesions are not common. But it is easy to forget that such a lesion may be tuberculous (p 72), even when the nearest lymph nodes are enlarged.

1.2 The changes after infection

1.2.1 The primary complex. When the tiny drops carrying the bacilli are breathed in they are carried through the air passages to just under the surface of the lung.

There they remain and the TB slowly multiply in numbers. As that happens some are carried in the lymph to the nearest lymph nodes beside the bronchi. In both places the presence of the bacilli causes a reaction and the defence cells of the body begin to collect. In about 4–8 weeks there is a small area at the centre of this process where the host tissues are dead (**caseation**) and around that area is an increasing ring of defence cells.

About this time most people become sensitive to tubercle bacilli, as shown by a **positive tuberculin skin test** (p 200).

The changes in the lung and in the lymph nodes are together known as the **Primary Complex** (Figure 8).

From that time the result depends upon the power of the child to resist the multiplication of the bacilli and limit the amount of caseation.

That power varies with age (p 11), being least in the very young. It also varies with nutrition. Poor nutrition lowers body defences (p 11).

Most people manage, slowly over many months, to heal both the focus in the lung and that in the lymph nodes.

But it takes time and TB can remain inactive but living and capable of multiplication for many years (Figure 3, p 9).

From the time of infection bacilli escape into the **bloodstream** and are carried to other parts of the body. Fortunately disease does not always result (see p 35 below).

The risk may be small for any individual child. But in a community where there are many adults spreading infection many children will become ill.

We must now look at the changes which occur when the infection progresses and the child becomes ill.

1.2.2 *Rupture of focus into the pleural space (Figure 8b).* We have seen that the primary focus forms just below the surface of the lung. Most do not become larger than 10 mm. Sometimes the focus does get bigger still. Then the surface of the lung may rupture allowing caseous material and sometimes bacilli to leak into the pleural space.

The result seems to depend on the child's nutrition and degree of tuberculin sensitivity. When nutrition is good and sensitivity is strong much fluid is produced and a large effusion results. When sensitivity is low in the young or malnourished child the reaction is much less.

The fluid of an effusion is usually absorbed without difficulty. But occasionally if many bacilli are present the fluid may become purulent and a **tuberculous empyema** is the result.

1.2.3 *Acute cavitation of focus (Figure 8c).* When resistance is poor as in young or malnourished children the primary focus may increase in size. Instead of leaking into the pleural space it may open into a small bronchus and the caseous material is discharged by coughing.

During this process there may be a stage when air can enter the small

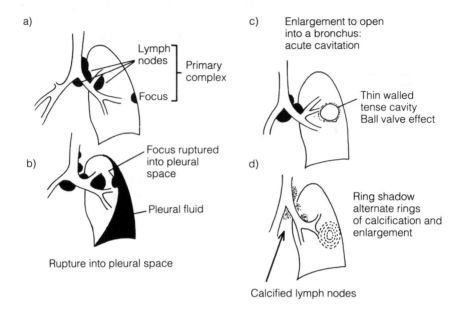

Figure 8 *Complications of primary tuberculous complex.* **a) Primary lesion** in left lung. The lung component is often quite a faint shadow on the X-ray. Note the enlarged hilum and paratracheal lymph nodes. (The drawing is diagrammatic: in an X-ray the shadows are usually less well-defined.) **b) Pleural effusion** produced by a rupture of the lung component of the primary complex. (In an X-ray the lung lesion is usually hidden by the effusion: this drawing is diagrammatic.) **c)** Thin-walled **cavity** resulting from rupture of primary lung lesion into a bronchus. Bacilli may spread from this cavity to other parts of the lung. **d)** Rounded **coin lesion** representing primary lung component. Later it may become calcified. At this stage, as shown, the hilar and paratracheal lymph nodes may also show calcification. As it calcifies, at some stage there may be rings of calcification around the lung lesion, as we show here.

cavity when the patient is breathing in but cannot escape when he is breathing out. The result is the formation of a small thin-walled cavity.

This process can speed infection to other parts of the lungs. Spread may also occur by the erosion of the tuberculous nodes through the bronchial wall. Caseous material and TB from the nodes may then spread through the bronchi to other parts of the lung.

We have twice seen a child who suffocated from caseous material suddenly blocking both main bronchi. Emergency bronchoscopy, if available, could save such a child. If this is not available, we suggest turning the child upside down and percussing the chest with the open hand to try to help the child to cough up the material and clear the bronchi.

This type of progressive lung disease is particularly likely in malnourished children. It can proceed so rapidly that the child may die from tuberculous pneumonia before developing signs of blood spread disease such as miliary tuberculosis or tuberculous meningitis.

1.2.4 *Ring or coin shadow (Figure 8d).* Very occasionally in older children (and found only by X-ray examination) a round coin-like lesion can be seen in the lung field. Sometimes the edge is calcified or a series of zones of calcification may be seen representing periods of healing and extension. This can remain unchanged for long periods. It may then completely or partially calcify.

1.2.5 *The lymph nodes at the root of the lung (Figures 9–16).* Bacilli from the primary focus reach the lymph nodes by direct drainage. These nodes lie near to the air passages (bronchi). Both the nodes and the air passages get larger towards the centre (root) of the lung.

The bacilli in the nodes cause a change which is the same as that in the focus in the lung and the node becomes larger and may soften.

In very young children the nodes can press upon and narrow the soft air passages and cause collapse of that part of the lung (Figures 9 and 10). In the older child a node can break through the wall of the bronchus.

When that happens the soft contents of the node can leak into the air passage and as the child breathes in the material containing bacilli can be drawn further into the lung. So the disease is spread (Figure 11, p 35).

This is a common method of spread in young poorly nourished children.

If the child's defences are better, there is merely an **extensive exudate** of fluid and cells into that part of the lung. This is due to hypersensitivity to the TB or to tuberculoprotein in the caseous material. This exudate, as seen on the X-ray, later clears completely (Figure 12, p 36).

Occasionally the contents of the lymph nodes are firmer and simply stick into the bronchus so that when the child breathes in, air can pass the narrowed space but when the child breathes out the gap is closed and the air is trapped ('obstructive emphysema') (Figure 13, p 37). This blows up the lung beyond the narrowing. In most cases this does not last very long. The block becomes complete and the lung beyond collapses.

Any of these forms of pneumonia, exudate or collapse may result in damage to the bronchi of the lobe or segment which may give rise to **bronchiectasis** (Figure 14, p 38).

1.2.6 *Other complications of lymph node disease.* So far the complications we have described have resulted from the lymph nodes damaging the bronchi. But two other structures in the chest may be affected.

There is a group of large lymph nodes in the space where the main windpipe (trachea) divides to supply a branch to each lung.

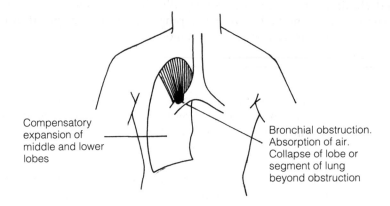

Compensatory
expansion of
middle and lower
lobes

Bronchial obstruction.
Absorption of air.
Collapse of lobe or
segment of lung
beyond obstruction

Figure 9   *Complications of mediastinal lymph nodes of primary complex:* **collapse of right upper lobe** with expansion of middle and lower lobes to compensate

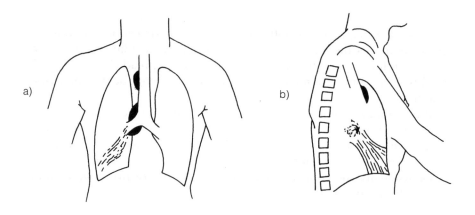

a)

b)

Figure 10   *Complications of mediastinal lymph nodes of primary complex:* **collapse of middle lobe** of right lung. The nature of the shadow is much clearer in a lateral X-ray film (b)

At the front this group is in close contact with the back of the pericardium which surrounds the heart. At the back they are near the gullet as it goes down to pass through the diaphragm to the stomach.

If this group of nodes enlarges and softens with tuberculosis it may involve the pericardium. The node contents may leak into the pericardium producing a **pericardial effusion** (Figure 15, p 39). (See also

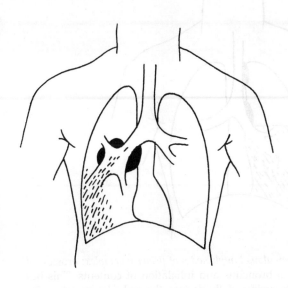

Contents of lymph
node leak into bronchus

Sucked into lung beyond
the leak

If many TB, causes
tuberculous bronchopneumonia.
This may cause lung
destruction or healing
with contraction

Figure 11 *Complications of mediastinal lymph nodes of primary complex:* erosion (bursting) of mediastinal lymph nodes into a bronchus. The material has been sucked into a bronchus beyond the leak. This has led to **tuberculous broncho-pneumonia**. The bronchopneumonia may cause lung destruction or healing with contraction (shrinkage) of the lung

p 118.) Very occasionally, instead of reaching to the front the mass of nodes becomes attached to the **gullet** (oesophagus).

1.2.7 Blood spread of bacilli (Figure 16, p 40). During the time the primary complex is forming and for some time afterwards bacilli escape into the bloodstream from both the focus and the nodes. This may occur either by eroding a blood vessel in the lesion or through the lymphatics.

The bloodstream carries the TB to distant parts of the body such as liver, spleen, bones, brain and kidneys. This process ceases as the child heals the primary focus and its nodes but it can continue for many months. Most of these bacilli although they form small tubercles do not cause any clinical illness and are healed by the child's own defensive powers.

But in very young children defences are weak. They are also reduced by malnutrition or by other infectious diseases, particularly measles and whooping cough, in some countries by HIV infection. In these children primary infection may be rapidly followed by **miliary tuberculosis** and/or **tuberculous meningitis**. These are still fatal diseases if not properly treated. If the child's defences are better, or fewer bacilli spread, one of

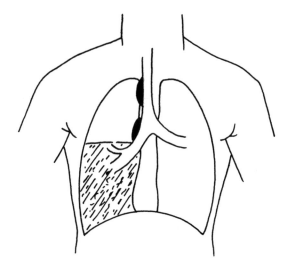

Figure 12 *Complications of tuberculous lymph nodes of primary complex:* erosion of tuberculous lymph nodes into a bronchus and inhalation of contents. This has caused extensive **exudate** (outpouring of fluid) into the right lower lobe. The child may be much less ill than the X-ray appearances might suggest. The shadow may clear slowly but completely over a number of months. On the X-ray alone you cannot distinguish this shadow from a very extensive tuberculous pneumonia. But with a tuberculous pneumonia the child would be much more ill. Both are different from an acute bacterial pneumonia which comes on quickly and improves with an antibiotic. The large hilar and paratracheal nodes on the X-ray make tuberculosis much more probable.

the more chronic lesions may show after months or years. These include tuberculosis of **bones, joints, kidneys** etc.

Any of these lesions, including miliary or meningitis, may occur at any time in life if there is a dormant (sleeping) lesion somewhere in the body and the patient's resistance is lowered.

Tuberculosis of the **cervical lymph nodes** is common in Africa and Asia. In Europe this was most frequently due to bovine bacilli acquired from milk. The primary lesion (often invisible) was in the tonsil or mouth. The lymph node component was in the draining nodes in the upper part of the neck. Bovine TB have not been found in man in India, and are probably rare elsewhere in Asia. In these areas it seems probable that the disease, at least in the nodes above the clavicle, is due to spread from intrathoracic lymph nodes associated with a primary lesion in the lung. The frequency of bovine infection in Africa is still uncertain (p 7).

Peritoneal tuberculosis is also common in high prevalence countries. Where milk infection is rare, it must either be due to food contamination with TB or to blood spread.

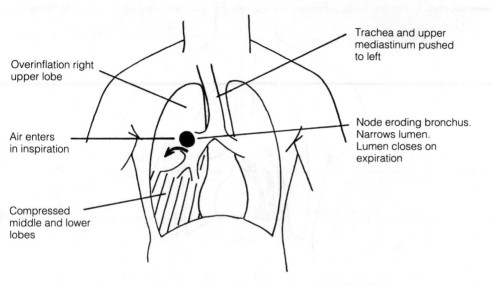

Trachea and upper
mediastinum pushed
to left

Overinflation right
upper lobe

Air enters
in inspiration

Node eroding bronchus.
Narrows lumen.
Lumen closes on
expiration

Compressed
middle and lower
lobes

Figure 13 *Complications of tuberculous lymph nodes of primary complex:* ball valve obstruction of the upper lobe bronchus by an enlarged hilar lymph node. This allows air in, but not out, of the right upper lobe. The right upper lobe is blown up (distended) by '**obstructive emphysema**'. Note the compressed middle and lower lobes, and that the trachea is pushed to the opposite side. On the X-ray the inflated area looks blacker than the rest of the lung and has few lung markings

SOME STORIES ABOUT PRIMARY TUBERCULOSIS AND ITS COMPLICATIONS

A family outbreak of tuberculosis

A family of a father, mother, two boys aged 7 and 3, and a baby girl of 9 months, lived in a provincial town. The **boy, Ong, aged 3** became **vaguely unwell**. He had a **low fever**. Sometimes he ate a meal normally, **sometimes he refused all food**. His mother took him to a local doctor. The doctor found nothing definite, but gave him penicillin.

After 7–10 days, Ong began to **vomit**. The doctor sent him to the District Hospital, where he was admitted. **On examination** he was fretful, thin and rather dry. There were no other abnormal physical signs. **X-ray of chest** showed enlargement of shadows at the left lung root. **Tuberculin test** with 2 TU showed 8 mm induration in 48 hours. **Lumbar puncture** showed 186 cells per mm³ and 100 mg protein per cent. (Culture later grew TB.) This, with the X-ray, strongly suggested **tuberculous meningitis**. **Treatment** was immediately started: he made a complete recovery. When the diagnosis was made, the **family was examined**. Father's sputum was

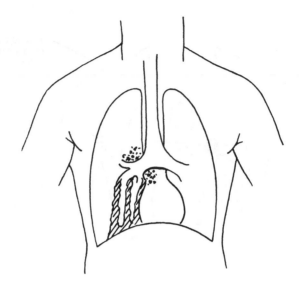

Figure 14 *Complications of tuberculous lymph nodes of primary complex:* **bronchiectasis** in a collapsed right lower lobe due to an old tuberculous primary complex. Calcification of hilar lymph nodes (showing more intensely white on the X-ray) suggest the cause of the collapse. Because the lower lobe bronchus is poorly drained by gravity there is often secondary infection and symptoms of bronchiectasis. The same may occur in the middle lobe

negative. **Mother's sputum was positive**. Her X-ray chest showed extensive tuberculosis.

The **brother, Sak, aged 7** was found to be **unwell, listless**, and with a slight **cough. Tuberculin test** was positive. **X-ray of chest** showed a primary complex on the right side. He rapidly improved with **treatment**.

The **baby girl, Shinta, then aged 9 months**, was tuberculin negative. Because of contact with the mother, BCG was not given at once. The **tuberculin test** was **repeated** after 1 month. It was then strongly positive. She was therefore also treated.

All the family took their treatment regularly. All made a complete recovery. Some years later, chest X-rays of all three children showed a calcified primary complex.

Comment: This family was very well managed. When the first child's illness did not improve with penicillin, the doctor referred him to hospital. The hospital doctor realised the child was ill and admitted him. He then thought of the possibility of tuberculosis. This was confirmed by the X-ray and tuberculin test. The lumbar puncture showed that there

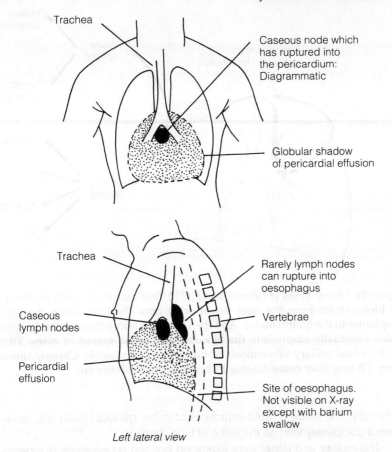

Trachea

Caseous node which
has ruptured into
the pericardium:
Diagrammatic

Globular shadow
of pericardial effusion

Trachea

Rarely lymph nodes
can rupture into
oesophagus

Caseous
lymph nodes

Vertebrae

Pericardial
effusion

Site of oesophagus.
Not visible on X-ray
except with barium
swallow

Left lateral view

Figure 15 *Complications of tuberculous lymph nodes of primary complex:* **pericardial effusion** due to rupture of a tuberculous lymph node into the pericardium. We show the lymph node in the diagram but you would not see it in the X-ray

was early meningitis. The doctor then went on to examine the family. So he diagnosed and cured three other family members.

Primary tuberculosis with bronchial erosion

A girl, Sandra, aged 4 years was an only child. Her mother took her to hospital because she was **losing weight** and had had a **cough** for about 2 months. On **examination** she looked **thin**. There was a suspicion that the **left side of the chest** did not move as well as the right; the air entry on that side was reduced. She could not produce any sputum. Her **tuberculin test** was strongly positive. **X-ray** showed scattered areas of patchy shadowing throughout the left lung and some enlargement of the root of the lung. The doctor started Sandra on anti-tuberculosis chemo-

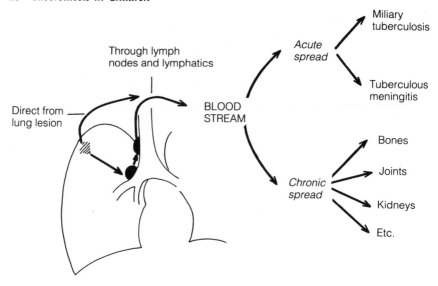

Figure 16   *Blood spread of tubercle bacilli* (TB) This can occur either a) directly to the bloodstream from the lung lesion or b) from the lung lesion through the lymphatics to the lymph nodes. And then from the nodes through the lymphatics which eventually empty into the bloodstream. **Acute spread** of many TB may result in fatal miliary tuberculosis or tuberculous meningitis. **Chronic spread** of fewer TB may later cause disease in bones, joints, kidneys etc

therapy. She made a rapid improvement in her general health and recovered completely with no evidence of lung damage.

The mother and father were examined but had no evidence of tuberculosis. Sandra often visited a **grandmother**. The mother said 'Yes, the grandmother had a chronic cough'. She was brought up to hospital. There she was found to have TB in the sputum. In due course she was cured by treatment.

Comment: A story of 2 months' cough and loss of weight made pneumonia an unlikely diagnosis. Tuberculosis was more probable. The strongly positive tuberculin test, combined with the X-ray findings, made this diagnosis certain.

Collapse right middle and lower lobes due to caseous material from a tuberculous lymph node obstructing bronchi

A girl, Bimla, aged 12 began to feel ill while at school. She felt **feverish** and had a **headache**. She returned home. Her mother put her to bed where she developed a **dry cough**. A doctor saw her and gave her penicillin. She improved slightly for a few days, but then the cough and headache came back. The doctor sent her to the District Hospital where she was admitted.

On examination Bimla had a fever of 38.9°C. In the chest there was decreased movement of the right side. The heart and trachea were displaced to that side and the breath sounds greatly decreased. This suggested collapse of one or more lobes. **Chest X-ray** showed collapse of the right middle and lower lobes.

The hospital doctor at first gave Bimla penicillin. He also did a **tuberculin test**. In 48 hours this was strongly positive.

The doctor therefore changed the treatment to **antituberculosis chemotherapy**. Her fever at once began to come down.

There were no facilities for bronchoscopy at the hospital. Something was obstructing her right lower lobe and middle lobe bronchi. This might be caseous material coming from tuberculous lymph nodes. So the doctor tipped her, head down, over the side of the bed. He asked her to breathe deeply and cough hard while he rapidly percussed her right chest with his open hand. He asked the nurse to repeat this twice a day. During one of these treatments she started to have an acute fit of coughing. She coughed up some cheesy material. The doctor sent this for microscopy: TB were seen in it. After the fit of coughing Bimla's right chest moved better and both sides now seemed normal. Repeat X-ray showed that the lobes had re-expanded.

Bimla's temperature became normal in 10 days. She completed full treatment and remained well.

Her family were examined but no-one else was found to have tuberculosis.

1.3 The timetable and risks of primary infection (Figure 17)

Following the general statement given above we know something about the usual timetable of tuberculosis by long observation of European children whose time of infection was known. The common timetable of the complications of primary tuberculosis can be set out in a diagram (Figure 17). This diagram also gives some indication of the factors which increased the risk of the most serious complications. These risks were found in children in a well-nourished population before effective treatment was available. Risks are likely to be greater in any population where malnutrition or HIV infection is common. Figure 17 shows the time relationships of the development of the primary complex after the child has been infected, and that most go on to heal (1), but complications can arise from the focus in the lung (2), from the lymph nodes (3) and then spread to other organs, brain (4), bone (5) and much later the kidneys (6). It also gives an indication how long after infection complications are most likely to occur and of the things (7) which make a primary infection more dangerous by reducing the body's power to resist the multiplication of the tubercle bacilli.

Limited evidence from **Africa and Asia** suggests (surprisingly) that the latent period between primary infection and the development of

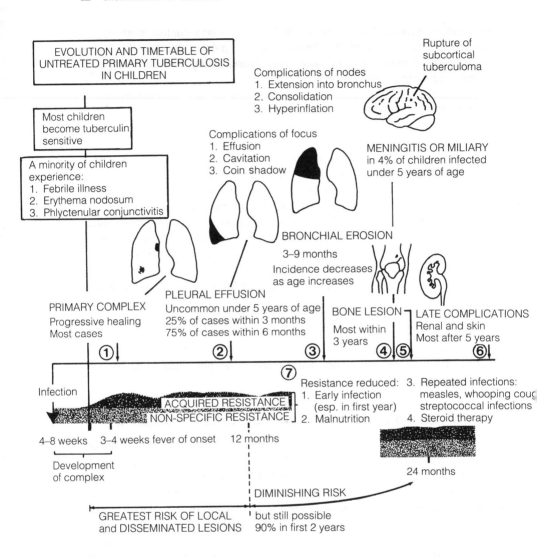

EVOLUTION AND TIMETABLE OF UNTREATED PRIMARY TUBERCULOSIS IN CHILDREN

Most children become tuberculin sensitive

A minority of children experience:
1. Febrile illness
2. Erythema nodosum
3. Phlyctenular conjunctivitis

Complications of nodes
1. Extension into bronchus
2. Consolidation
3. Hyperinflation

Rupture of subcortical tuberculoma

Complications of focus
1. Effusion
2. Cavitation
3. Coin shadow

MENINGITIS OR MILIARY in 4% of children infected under 5 years of age

BRONCHIAL EROSION

3–9 months
Incidence decreases as age increases

PRIMARY COMPLEX
Progressive healing
Most cases

PLEURAL EFFUSION
Uncommon under 5 years of age
25% of cases within 3 months
75% of cases within 6 months

BONE LESION
Most within 3 years

LATE COMPLICATIONS
Renal and skin
Most after 5 years

① ② ③ ④ ⑤ ⑥

⑦

Infection

ACQUIRED RESISTANCE
NON-SPECIFIC RESISTANCE

Resistance reduced:
1. Early infection (esp. in first year)
2. Malnutrition

3. Repeated infections: measles, whooping coug streptococcal infections
4. Steroid therapy

4–8 weeks   3–4 weeks fever of onset   12 months

24 months

Development of complex

DIMINISHING RISK

GREATEST RISK OF LOCAL and DISSEMINATED LESIONS

but still possible 90% in first 2 years

Figure 17 *Evolution and timetable of untreated primary tuberculous infection.* (Reproduced with permission from Miller, F.J.W. *Tuberculosis in Children*. New Delhi: Churchill-Livingstone, 1986.)

pulmonary tuberculosis in adult life is much longer than was found in Europe (see p 11). At present it is uncertain how far the timetable given in Figure 17 applies to developing countries.

1.4 The effect of age at infection, nutrition and other infections and infestations (See also p 11)

The power to resist infection is the power of the defences of the body to overcome an invading organism. This depends on the age of the person infected, upon his or her nutrition, upon the presence of other infections (especially HIV infection) or infestations and upon the nature of the infection itself whether it acts suddenly like cholera or very slowly like leprosy.

In tuberculosis the bacilli grow slowly over weeks and months rather than days. So the effects and signs of the disease appear slowly.

The changes which follow the first infection have been given above. We also showed how most of those who have a first infection with tuberculosis manage to heal it. Their bodies have indeed learned to respond more quickly to future attacks by TB. If they should get another infection the body's quicker defence prevents the spread of bacilli to other organs, as occurs during the first infection.

This is the reason why **BCG**, a harmless form of primary infection, reduces the frequency of miliary tuberculosis and tuberculous meningitis.

But the defences do not work so well at every **age**. They are poor at birth and improve slowly for the first 10 years or so of life. **Up to puberty** the child is not so good at preventing **blood spread**, though this gradually improves with age. But a well nourished child seems good at preventing the spread of disease **within the lung** itself. **After puberty** the body is better at preventing blood spread, but much poorer at preventing spread in the lungs. But badly nourished children may develop severe cavitating lung disease at an early age.

Throughout life the body only responds to infection in the best way if it is well nourished with an adequate supply of the proper food.

At any age insufficient food, leading to **malnutrition**, reduces the power of the body to respond to its full capacity. This increases not only the seriousness of disease but also the number of deaths.

The other factor which reduces resistance to tuberculosis is the presence of **other infections**. In children this seems especially so with measles and whooping cough for if they occur while the child has a primary infection with tuberculosis that disease may extend and miliary tuberculosis or meningitis develops. In some areas of the world HIV infection is the most important other infection (p 82).

Severe **worm infestation**, particularly with intestinal parasites, can be a cause of malnutrition, particularly if the amount of food taken is only just enough.

2: MEETING THE CHILD WHO MIGHT HAVE TUBERCULOSIS

2.1 When to think of tuberculosis (and see Section 3 p 50 for more detail)

It is not enough to understand how children are infected with tuberculosis or how the disease may spread. You must also know when to think that a child who comes to see you may have the disease. Remember to think of it whenever you see a child who is thin or has:

1. **Failed to gain weight** or has lost weight for more than 4 weeks (a weight chart is valuable).
2. **Lost energy** and possibly some weight over 2–3 months.
3. Either (1) or (2) as described above but also with a **wheeze** or **cough** which may occasionally seem like whooping cough.
4. Has had a **fever** or raised temperature more than a week without any explanation.
5. Any or all of (1), (2), (3) and the **sign of fluid** – dullness, on one side of the chest.
6. A **swollen abdomen**, especially if there is any lump to be felt and if the lump remains after treatment for worms.
7. A child with **chronic diarrhoea** with large white stools which has not responded to treatment for worms or giardiasis (with metronidazole).
8. A **limp on walking**; a **stiff spine** and is unwilling to bend his or her back.
9. **Spinal hump** with or without stiffness in walking.
10. **Swelling of knee** or ankle, wrist, elbow or shoulder, rib or **any bone or joint** which is not due to injury.
11. A swollen, painless, firm or soft, **lymph node** swelling sometimes with smaller lymph nodes near to it and sometimes matted to it.
12. A **lymph node abscess** which may be affecting or coming through the skin.
13. One or more **soft swellings under the skin**. They are not painful. The skin may have broken leaving an ulcer with sharply cut edges and usually a clean base.
14. A **discharging sinus** (wound) near any joint.
15. **Headache and irritability**, occasional vomiting, child wishes to be left alone and gradually becomes less rousable over 2–3 weeks.
16. **Slow onset of weakness** in one arm or leg or side of face.

2.2 Important points to remember

1. Tuberculosis and **malnutrition** go together: tuberculosis can cause kwashiorkor or xerophthalmia or vitamin B deficiency.
2. The slow onset of **typhoid** (enteric) fever or paratyphoid can be like tuberculosis.
3. **Chronic infections** of the nose and lungs may be present at the same time as tuberculosis.
4. **Malaria** and tuberculosis may be present together in the same child or one may be mistaken for the other.
5. Swellings of lymph nodes such as **lymphoma** can resemble tuberculosis.
6. Your patient may have **more than one infection** or infestation and different parasites are found in different regions – what types have you in your locality?
7. Particularly in Africa and SE Asia it may be necessary to consider whether a child may have tuberculosis complicating **HIV infection**. This may be congenital or acquired from a contaminated needle or through an open wound contaminated by someone's blood. AIDS in children may closely resemble tuberculosis (see p 83).

2.3 How to plan action – recording of a child suspected to be tuberculous

Always be ready to SUSPECT **tuberculosis**. Record information and results of examination systematically as follows. (Preferably use any standard tuberculosis records for children produced by your national tuberculosis programme: see also 'Plan of action' p 47)

1. **Names** of patient, father and mother.
2. **Address** or location of house.
3. **Age** and **sex** of patient.
4. **Weight** and **height**; weight for age, 'Road to Health Chart'.
5. **BCG**, history of injection, presence of scar – yes/no.
6. **Family history** of tuberculosis, or suggestive of tuberculosis. Remember the grandparent with a chronic cough. Remember to ask about relatives who have died recently and had a cough.
7. **Duration** of present illness.
8. **Parents' complaint** concerning child: cough, sweat, loss of weight, appetite or energy, limp, change in behaviour or temper, headache, lumps or swellings.
9. **Child's symptoms and signs** found on examination:

    • Abdomen: pain, swelling, enlargement of spleen or liver.
    • Chest: cough, wheeze or pain. Any dullness to percussion suggesting consolidation or fluid.

- Limbs: swelling of joints, pain on walking, stiffness.
- Spine: stiffness or hump.
- Skin: ulcers or sores; swollen lymph nodes, neck groin or armpit.

An African child with tuberculosis often loses skin pigmentation. If the child's skin is paler than his mother's think of tuberculosis. But remember a child with kwashiorkor may also have a pale skin or that the father may be lighter skinned.

10. **Tuberculin test**. Although there may be difficulties in judging the results in any individual child, a test may be helpful (see Appendix E p 200). Read and record result in 48–72 hours. A positive result (see p 201) in a child with weight for age within the 'Road to Health' is significant. In a malnourished child, or a child with HIV infection, the test may be weak or negative even when there is active tuberculosis. The test may also be negative if the child is very ill, or wasted. This is especially so in miliary tuberculosis or tuberculous meningitis. In many countries weak positives may also occur from infection from common environmental mycobacteria which do not cause disease (p 7). Weak positives also occur after BCG. Therefore in a difficult case do a tuberculin test (p 200) if this is available. If the test is strongly positive (p 202), especially in a young child, this is strongly in favour of recent TB infection or clinical tuberculosis (though not conclusive proof). But a negative test in an ill or malnourished child is **not** against tuberculosis.

11. **X-ray**. Whenever possible obtain an X-ray of the chest and of any other suspicious area. You must consider the results in relation to all the other clinical evidence. Interpretation of children's X-rays can be difficult. We have tried to give some guidance in the notes on Figure 8 (p 32) and Figures 9–15 (p 34 and following). Where X-ray is not possible, you may have to make up your mind on clinical evidence alone.

12. Children do not usually produce **sputum**. But if they do it should be examined for TB by microscopy. The same applies to any other fluid obtainable. If you cannot do it on the spot, you can send suitable specimens to the nearest large hospital or laboratory. This will depend on your local organisation.

13. In a well equipped hospital you may be able to arrange for a **gastric suction** specimen for culture for TB. This investigation is distressing for the child. Only do it if you think it is essential, e.g. when the diagnosis is particularly difficult. For details see Appendix F p 206).

14. When you suspect tuberculosis, if you can, send the child to a centre where full investigation is possible. But we realise in many places this may not be possible. In that case you will find guidance on p 47) below.

15. NB It is now of particular importance to avoid the spread of HIV:

whenever possible do not re-use needles. If possible do not re-use syringes. If they must be re-used make sure they are properly sterilised (needle **and** syringe) between patients.

In areas where **child malnutrition** is common and the risk of infection is high the primary infection in the lung and lymph nodes often goes on to progressive disease. So more children come with chest complaints and loss of weight and energy. But tuberculosis does not always cause dramatic physical signs in the lungs.

Cough is usually soft. **Wheeze** (due to lymph node pressure on bronchi) is gentle, heard both when breathing in and out. Children very rarely **spit blood**. (When they do it may be due to whooping cough.) The child's **temperature** may be raised, but very high temperatures are not common. If you suspect trouble in the chest and the child cannot be moved to a larger hospital, then it is necessary to do the very best you can. If you can, get the child X-rayed. When you see the film you must judge it together with all the other information about the child. This includes the length of the history of the illness, the appearance of the child, the physical signs and the family history (known tuberculosis or possible tuberculosis), and the results of the tuberculin test (if available).

The following make it more likely that you are **not dealing with tuberculosis** but with another bacterial infection: a) short history of illness, b) loud physical signs in the chest, c) acutely ill child and d) no history suggestive of possible tuberculosis in family or neighbours.

The following makes it more likely that you **are dealing with tuberculosis**: a) illness already for some weeks, b) child chronically rather than acutely ill, c) few physical signs, d) a family history of known or possible tuberculosis and e) a strongly positive tuberculin test. Look also for signs of tuberculosis in other parts of the body (p 55 and following).

2.4 Plan of action

When you cannot yourself make a definite diagnosis and when you cannot refer the patient to a large hospital you will have to take action yourself. A 'score chart' is very useful. Several have been developed and used. They help by bringing together the clinical evidence and by giving different values to the various pieces of information. One of these score charts which has been developed and used for some years in Papua New Guinea has proved very useful. We are grateful to Dr Keith Edwards for permission to reproduce this chart. It consists of two parts. First a **Score Chart (A)** (Table 3) to summarise the results of your history taking, observation and examination. When this has been completed

Table 3   *Paediatric tuberculosis score chart A (Courtesy of Dr Keith Edwards, University of Papua New Guinea)*

Patients details	Hospital or PHC location
Name	
Age yrs	Date
(d.o.b. / /)	Scored by;
Sex M/F	
Weight kg	Nurse Health Ass. Doctor
BCG scars 0/1/2/3	

SCORE CHART (Circle box and write in score)
Children suspected to have tuberculosis

Feature	0	1	3	SCORE
LENGTH OF ILLNESS	LESS THAN 2 WEEKS	2–4 WEEKS	MORE THAN 4 WEEKS	
NUTRITION (WEIGHT)	ABOVE 80% FOR AGE	BETWEEN 60% and 80%	LESS THAN 60%	
FAMILY TUBERCULOSIS PAST OR PRESENT	NONE	REPORTED BY FAMILY	PROVED SPUTUM POSITIVE	

SCORE FOR OTHER FEATURES IF PRESENT

Positive tuberculin test	3	
Large painless lymph nodes; firm, soft, sinus in neck, axilla, groin	3	
Unexplained fever, night sweats, no response to malaria treatment	2	
Malnutrition, not improving after 4 weeks	3	
Angle deformity of spine	4	
Joint swelling, bone swelling or sinuses	3	
Unexplained abdominal mass or ascites	3	
CNS: change in temperament fits or coma (send to hospital if possible)	3	

TOTAL SCORE

When score is 7 or more treat for TB – see notes

you are left with a score for the patient varying from zero (0) to seven or more.

The second **part (B)** (Figure 18) is a **Flow Chart** depending upon the score and whether the patient has signs of a pneumonia which has lasted more than 2 weeks. If the score is 7 or more you are justified in beginning anti-tuberculosis treatment immediately and watching the patient very closely. With effective chemotherapy you usually see improvement very quickly.

If the score is less than 7 and the patient has signs of chest infection (pneumonia) then give a broad spectrum antibiotic and follow the flow chart as indicated in B.

Use of plans A and B. When a child comes with a chest illness and signs of pneumonia, there may not be enough evidence to show its cause. First use the **Score Chart A** (Table 3). Then use the pathways shown by the direction of arrows in **Flow Chart B** (Figure 18). The first step is to fill in the **Score Chart A** (Table 3) giving the points as shown in the two boxes (you will see that in order to do this there must be a careful history

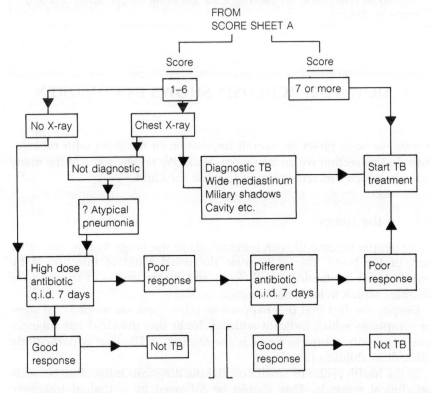

Details of types and doses of antibiotics etc., given in Section 4

Figure 18 *Paediatric tuberculosis Flow Chart B* (Courtesy of Dr Keith Edwards, University of Papua New Guinea) For use when presentation suggests pneumonia and there are no other signs of tuberculosis

and clinical examination). Scores are given **only** for findings which can be answered at the time of the examination.

If the score is 7 or more start tuberculosis treatment. If the score is 1–6, if possible get an X-ray of the chest.

If there is **no X-ray**, treat with antibiotics for 7 days and note response. If response poor, change the antibiotic and treat for another 7 days. After that second week, if there is still no response begin treatment for tuberculosis.

If there is an X-ray, and the diagnosis is still doubtful, follow the path described in Flow Chart B. If the X-ray suggests tuberculosis begin treatment for it. (For details of treatment see p 76.)

IMPORTANT NOTE

This plan of treatment will only succeed if you observe the patient closely. Record all changes in his behaviour, temperature, weight, symptoms and signs of disease.

3: HOW TUBERCULOSIS SHOWS IN CHILDREN

Above we have given an overall impression of the child with tuberculosis. In this section we go into more detail. We review some of the many ways in which tuberculosis may show in the child.

3.1   In the lungs

More people become ill with tuberculosis in the lungs than in any other part of the body. This is because the usual route of infection is by breathing air containing bacilli (p 9) and the extension of the primary complex which follows the infection (p 30).

Despite the fact that this happens so often there are no physical signs or symptoms which indicate without doubt that the child has tuberculosis. The only complete proof is the finding of TB. That is particularly difficult in children (p 46).

In the health centre or small hospital the diagnosis must often be made on clinical grounds. This should be followed by a trial of treatment with careful observation. So in these conditions the **history** and **clinical examination** become all important. It is well worth while taking time and trouble over the history, which is often the most important clue to the diagnosis. Listen carefully to what the mother says. If there are signs or symptoms of illness this usually indicates that the tuberculosis is extending. The extension may be in the focus in the lung, in the lymph nodes into which the focus drains, or in the body generally (p 35).

When first seen the complaint is frequently that the child has lost or failed to gain **weight** or that he has **lost his normal energy** and activity. He may **sweat** and may have a **cough** and/or a **mild wheeze**. But the cough is usually unproductive so that sputum is hard to get. Children with tuberculosis practically never cough blood or blood-stained spit. All this has usually been present for some weeks before the child is brought to be seen.

There may be signs of vitamin deficiency. These may have appeared either before or after the general change in health was noticed.

The **family history** is important. Do the parents or grandparents have any history of cough or have they had any treatment for tuberculosis? Are any neighbours known to have a chronic cough or tuberculosis? Sometimes a family history of tuberculosis may be suppressed. Have there been any recent deaths in the family?

When you **examine** the child you must adapt yourself to his age. Young children will usually be nursed or held by one or other parent. Older children may stand or lie on a bed.

Always remember that you may **learn far more by watching carefully** than by any other way.

Train yourself to watch his behaviour, his physique (height and weight by age), his **skin** and **hair**, his **breathing** (remember he may be frightened).

Is there a **wheeze**, does he **cough** and if so is the cough loud or soft?

Does his **chest** move equally on both sides?

Does he seem to have any **pain on breathing** or elsewhere? If you tap his chest with your finger can you feel any difference on one side or the other – is there **dullness** which may show that there is fluid or solid lung in that area?

If you listen with a stethoscope can you detect if more air is entering one side of his chest than the other or can you hear a **wheeze** as when there is narrowing of the air passages?

Sometimes you will hear moist or wet **sounds** if there is fluid in the air passages.

But you must remember that whatever physical signs you find they only help you to understand what is happening in one or both lungs in a mechanical sense. **The signs do not tell you the cause of the changes**. Every piece of information must be considered and that is where the Score Sheet A (Table 3, p 48) can be a great help and the plan of action set out in Flow Chart B (Figure 18) can guide what you do (p 49).

3.1.1 Miliary tuberculosis. Miliary tuberculosis is the result of heavy blood spread of bacilli which then seed into lungs, liver, spleen and brain. At first only loss of energy and activity, loss of weight and fever are caused. There may not be any signs in the chest until the disease is far advanced. But X-ray of the chest, if this is possible, may show miliary shadows dotted throughout both lungs. This may not be obvious in the early stages. If it is not, try shining a very bright light behind the outer part of the intercostal spaces. This may pick up the small early shadows. (For a fuller discussion of miliary tuberculosis see p 107.)

THREE STORIES ABOUT MILIARY TUBERCULOSIS

Jumbe

A **boy**, Jumbe, **aged 6 months** was brought to hospital by his mother. She said that for a month or more he had had a **cough**. He was **losing weight**. Occasionally he **vomited**. Two weeks previously the baby's **right ear** began to **discharge**. About the same time she noticed **lumps** on both sides of his neck. They did not seem painful.

The doctor asked about the family. The mother then said that 3 months before the **father** had been admitted to hospital with **pulmonary tuberculosis**. At that time the child's **tuberculin test** was **negative**. He had not been given BCG. He had not seen his father since.

On **examination** the baby was alert but had obviously **lost weight**. The external meatus of the **right ear** was filled with **granulation tissue**. The skin was **ulcerated**. There were several **enlarged lymph nodes** on each side of the neck. The anterior **fontanelle** felt full. The doctor found **nothing abnormal in the lungs**. The **liver** was enlarged 2 finger-breadths below the costal margin. With his history, the doctor thought **tuberculosis** was likely. **X-ray of the chest** showed **miliary tuberculosis**.

Lumbar puncture showed 9 lymphocytes per mm³ and 65 mg of protein per cent in the cerebrospinal fluid (CSF). *TB* were seen in the CSF and in the discharge from the ear.

Treatment was begun at once. For the next week Jumbe was difficult to feed. He vomited occasionally. His abdomen became rather distended and the doctor could feel a **mass across the upper abdomen**.

But then, with treatment, Jumbe **gradually improved**. By the 4th month the mass could no longer be felt. The neck nodes remained small and firm. He made a complete recovery except that he was left with a **perforated eardrum**. X-ray at a year showed extensive calcification in the abdomen and the neck but the chest was normal, with no calcification.

Comment. The father had obviously infected Jumbe. But when the father was diagnosed Jumbe's **tuberculin test** had not yet become positive: the test should have been repeated 4–6 weeks later. If positive, but no evidence of illness, he should have been given chemoprophylaxis with isoniazid (p 197). If the test was negative he should have been given BCG. By getting the family history the hospital doctor immediately made the right diagnosis and treated the abdominal, ear, miliary and early tuberculous meningitis successfully.

Koresi

Koresi was just 2 years old when his mother first brought him to hospital. He was an only son. His mother's first child had died of whooping cough aged 5 months. Koresi had been watched at a clinic in his village from birth. He had gained weight well in his first 6 months but then more slowly. In his second year he was away from his own village. At about 18 months of age he **lost weight slowly**. He had **attacks of fever**, **cough** and **diarrhoea**. Finally, just at the end of his second year, his mother brought him to hospital.

His **tuberculin reaction** was **strongly positive**. His **X-ray** showed widespread **miliary tuberculosis**. He responded well to treatment. The source of infection was not found.

Koresi had been followed from birth: see weight chart (Figure 19). Note the loss of weight in the months before diagnosis and the rapid gain after treatment was started.

Imam

Lymph node tuberculosis and **miliary lesions** of lungs and skin. Imam, a twin boy aged 4, had been **vaguely unwell** since an attack of measles 8 months before. Then one day his mother found a **painless swelling above the inner end of his right clavicle**. She had also noticed that he had had several **crops of tiny, painless, non-irritable spots on his face, body and limbs**. The swelling in his neck then became soft and **discharged** some creamy pus. He was sent to hospital.

On **examination** Imam's general condition appeared good and his temperature was normal. In the right neck above the clavicle there was a **swelling** with a **central softening**. A small firm node was found on the left side also. There were many **small rather scaly spots** scattered over his body and limbs. They seemed to be in the skin and were about 1–3 mm in diameter. His **tuberculin reaction** was **strongly positive. X-ray** of his chest showed a partly calcified lesion in his right upper lobe, enlarged right paratracheal lymph nodes with early calcification and miliary tuberculosis. There was also calcification in the soft tissue swelling above his right clavicle. Pus was obtained from the abscess above the clavicle. Many TB were seen on direct examination.

On **treatment** the wound healed and both the skin lesions and the miliary lesions of the lungs disappeared. Imam made an uninterrupted recovery.

The **family** was examined. Both parents were healthy. His twin brother and elder sister were tuberculin negative. The source of his infection was unknown.

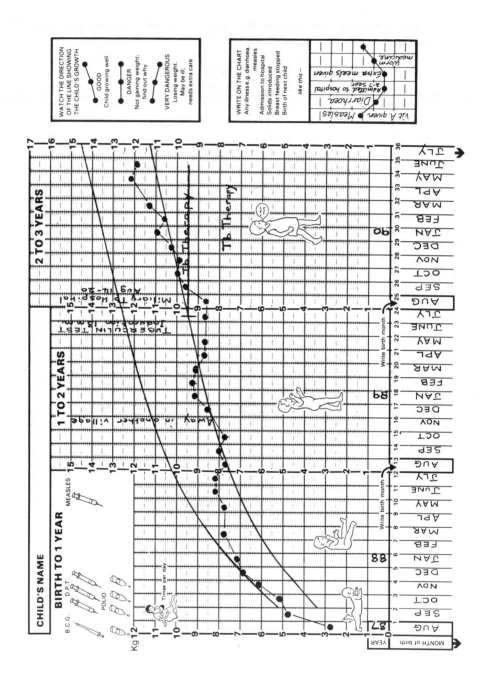

Figure 19 *Weight record* of a child with *miliary tuberculosis* in Western Nigeria (courtesy of Professor David Morley)

3.2   Infection in the mouth or ear

Although most children have their primary infection in the lungs and come to the health service with signs of chest disease, many get tuberculosis in other parts of the body. Also remember that the **primary infection can occur anywhere** on the skin or on any mucous membrane where bacilli can lodge.

Nearly always when that happens the first sign is painless swelling, and sometimes softening, of the **lymph nodes** draining the primary focus. If, for example, the focus is in the mouth or on a tonsil the nodes in the neck which drain the area become enlarged.

The **ear** or **mastoid** process can become infected in three ways.

1. Bacilli may be swept up the Eustachean tube when an infant or young child is feeding. The focus may then be inside the ear and the **node** is between the mastoid process and the angle of the jaw. The **ear runs**. The facial nerve may be involved so that the face on that side seems flat.
2. If that happens in a child who has already had a primary infection in some other site, there is still a chronic discharge from the ear but no enlarged node.
3. The **mastoid** may also become tuberculous by blood spread from a primary focus in the chest.

With any chronic painless discharge from the ear suspect tuberculosis. Get some of the material examined for TB (see case history on p 52).

3.3   Abdominal tuberculosis

Abdominal tuberculosis in children can begin in three ways:

1. from the milk of tuberculous cows that has been given to the child without previous boiling;
2. from foods or liquids, spoons or fingers which carry human bacilli from an adult who is coughing up large numbers and does not take proper care about when or where he coughs;
3. possibly through blood spread to the peritoneum from a primary focus in the lung.

Children very rarely get intestinal ulceration complicating their chest disease.

The **primary lesion** may be in the intestine and the nodes in the mesentery. The nodes enlarge, can soften and may leak their tuberculous contents into the abdominal cavity. The result is free fluid (**ascites**) and a **swollen abdomen**. In other cases the nodes, instead of rupturing, stick together the coils of the intestines. This can cause **pain** and **attacks of obstruction** which may even become complete. As the intestines become stuck to each other they may form **masses** which can be felt through the abdominal wall.

Tuberculosis can also spread to the pelvis and in girls involve the **fallopian tubes** and the **ovaries** so that the patient later becomes sterile. Abdominal tuberculosis is a common cause of later **infertility**.

You must distinguish swelling of the abdomen due to tuberculosis from other causes such as stretching of weak muscles in malnutrition or intestinal infestation. For details of abdominal tuberculosis in adults see p 128.

A PATIENT WITH ABDOMINAL TUBERCULOSIS

His parents brought **Wong aged 9** to hospital. For about 6 months he had been **vaguely unwell**. He had a **poor appetite** and occasional attacks of **right-sided abdominal pain**. For the past few days his symptoms had increased. His doctor had found his **temperature** was 39°C.

Wong's **parents** were healthy but an aunt had been found to have **pulmonary tuberculosis** 4 months earlier.

On **examination** his **abdomen** was somewhat distended and he was rather tender on the right side. Liver and spleen could not be felt. His **tuberculin test** was negative. **X-ray** of chest and abdomen was normal. No occult blood was found in the faeces.

For 3 days he remained unchanged and still running a fever. By the third day there was evidence of **free fluid in the abdomen**.

By the fifth day without a diagnosis the doctor decided to treat the illness as abdominal tuberculosis in spite of the negative tuberculin test. Within 48 hours of starting treatment Wong began to improve. His temperature began to fall, he began to eat and his abdominal swelling was less. After this he made a steady recovery. A tuberculin test was repeated after 2 months and was positive. He completed treatment and remained well.

3.4   Tuberculosis of the lymph nodes

3.4.1 *How it arises.* This is common. Most often the nodes in the neck are affected but sometimes those in the armpits or in the groin are affected. When that happens there is reason to think that there is a primary focus in the area which drains into the swollen nodes. You should look carefully for it. In other cases the cervical nodes above the clavicle are involved through spread by the lymphatics from the mediastinal nodes; the primary focus is in the lung. In a child with AIDS you may find lymph nodes enlarged throughout the body.

3.4.2 *How it shows in the patient.* The enlargement of the nodes is usually slow and painless. Children may be seen in three groups, depending on the state of the nodes:

1. The first group comes soon after the nodes have been found to be enlarged. There is one **large node** and several smaller ones near to it. The skin is not involved and the node feels firm.
2. The second group comes later when the nodes are matted together and the skin is fixed over them. These nodes are then becoming soft to form **abscesses** which will come through the skin and burst if they are not opened and the pus removed. The abscess is a 'cold' abscess. That is to say it is not hot or tender, but fluctuant (showing that it contains liquid).

    Draining the abscess through a small incision will preserve skin and result in a smaller scar as healing occurs with anti-tuberculosis treatment.
3. In the third group the nodes may **remain enlarged but firm** and may not soften for a considerable time after infection at a time when the child's resistance has been reduced by some other illness such as measles or whooping cough. But once that happens they behave like groups 1 and 2 described above and should be treated in the same way.

Generalised enlargement of the lymph nodes. In the past this was only very rarely due to tuberculosis. But in children with reduced immunity due to **HIV infection** a **primary infection with tuberculosis** may spread and cause general lymph node enlargement.

However, remember that general enlargement is often the first sign of **HIV infection itself**, even without tuberculosis. If in doubt, examine the mother, who may show evidence of AIDS.

Rarely it can also occur if a child with active AIDS is given **BCG**. The AIDS has reduced the child's immunity and allowed the BCG organisms to spread.

3.4.3 Diagnosing it from other conditions.

Nodes become infected for many other reasons and tuberculous nodes must be separated from:

1. **Acute septic inflammation**, in which the child is more acutely ill and the node swelling is rapid, painful and tender to touch. There is usually some septic lesion in the area drained by the node (perhaps hidden in the hair).
2. The firm smooth swelling of **Burkitt's lymphoma** arises from upper or lower jaw. It occurs in children in tropical Africa.
3. The swelling of **leukaemia**, usually generalised and with signs of bruising and anaemia.
4. In **lymphadenoma** the first nodes affected are usually just above the collar bone or in the armpit. They are painless and feel very hard. The spleen is often enlarged also.
5. Remember that the axillary (armpit) lymph nodes on the same side

often enlarge after **BCG vaccination**. Ask the mother and look for
the BCG scar.

You will often have to make the diagnosis purely on clinical grounds.
This is usually not difficult. In a difficult case insert a needle with
attached syringe into the node. Try to suck out material. Even if you get
no material, make a smear on a slide from the needle and stain for TB.
Culture if possible. Biopsy node if necessary (and available).

3.5   Tuberculosis of brain and spinal cord

Tuberculosis in the nervous system begins when TB spread through the
bloodstream, reach nervous tissue and local reaction forms a **tuberculoma**. This may cause symptoms because of its size, like a malignant
tumour. Or it may burst into the space surrounding the brain or spinal
cord and cause **meningitis**. The risk is greater and the diagnosis is more
difficult the younger the child.

3.5.1 Tuberculous meningitis (see also p 116).   When a tuberculoma in
the brain leaks or ruptures, living or dead bacilli escape into the surrounding space and around the base of the brain. There is a meningeal
reaction and the blood vessels in the base become involved. This reduces
the blood supply to the brain itself and finally, if there is no treatment,
blood supply stops. For treatment to be effective the illness must be
recognised and treated early and before there are signs of damage to the
brain.

Diagnosis is always urgent but the illness usually comes on gradually.
The condition must always be thought about when a previously happy
child becomes irritable. He may complain of headache or have vomiting
attacks. But the younger the child the greater the importance of change
in his usual behaviour.

Look particularly for resistance to flexing the neck forwards. Flexing
the knee and hip and then trying to extend the knee with the hip flexed
often results in the child extending his neck and back. Both these are
signs of '**meningism**', suggesting the possibility of meningitis, which
may be tuberculous. Look for signs of **cranial nerve lesions**, such as
squint (from sixth nerve paralysis) or weakness on one side of the face.
Look for possible **weakness of one side of the body**. Look for evidence
of **tuberculosis elsewhere** in the body, including an enlarged spleen
which might suggest miliary tuberculosis.

Tuberculous meningitis often complicates **miliary**, so that a chest X-
ray (if available) can be helpful. So can examination of the retina with
an ophthalmoscope if available. Dilate the pupils first. In a young irritable
child it may be necessary to give an anaesthetic in order to do a thorough
examination. But the presence of **choroidal tubercles** (p 71) is diagnostic.

If not diagnosed the child becomes more and more irritable and less responsive, wanting only to lie undisturbed. At that stage he often lies curled up on his side. The last stage of all is when he fails to respond to any rousing and lies on his back with outstretched stiff legs. From that stage there is little or no hope of recovery. The best hope is to see the child in the early stages. Unfortunately **infants** are often only brought to the doctor when they are **in coma**.

If you suspect tuberculous meningitis, when possible send the child to a hospital where X-ray, lumbar puncture and laboratory examination can be done. For details of laboratory findings and for diagnosis from other forms of meningitis see p 117 on tuberculous meningitis in adults.

If the transfer is not possible, then treatment must be started on suspicion but this should be avoided if at all possible. Details are given on p 176.

THREE PATIENTS WITH TUBERCULOUS MENINGITIS

Severe case: good recovery

Six weeks before admission to hospital Inez aged 20 months had an attack of **gastroenteritis** with loose stools and vomiting. She improved as the acute symptoms disappeared but she did not regain her normal health. Early one morning 3 weeks later she **vomited** and did so again several times the same day. For the next few days she was **irritable** and restless. She cried intermittently, especially at night when she would **wake screaming**. As time went on she grew steadily more irritable by day until, in the 3 days before admission, she had been **difficult to rouse**.

When Inez was aged 2 months she had had BCG vaccination because **her aunt had pulmonary tuberculosis**. But shortly afterwards her **mother** had also been found to have tuberculosis and had been admitted to hospital. The BCG had been given without separating Inez from her mother. She had probably been infected before she had been given the BCG.

On admission Inez was **febrile** (39°C), **drowsy** when left alone, **irritable** when handled. She had **lost weight**, there was **marked neck and back stiffness**. X-ray of the chest showed a **segmental lesion** in the left lower lobe and **early calcification** in the lymph nodes at the left hilum. The CSF contained 199 lymphocytes per mm³ and 140 mg protein per cent. No TB were seen on direct smear but they were later cultured.

Treatment was started immediately. During the first 10 days her condition did not change. On the 15th day she had **twitching movements** of her face and irregular jerking movements of arms and legs. These were controlled by increased sedation. For **2 months** more she lay quiet unless disturbed. But for increasing periods she seemed to become aware of her surroundings. She began to recognise her name. After **3 months** of treatment she was using words and in the next 3 months she learned to sit up, then stand

and finally to walk. At that time her CSF was normal. After that she made an uninterrupted recovery.

A child with tuberculosis of the submandibular lymph node followed by meningitis

Camilla age six had **toothache**. She then developed an **alveolar abscess** with a painful swelling of the **submandibular lymph node** draining the area. The tooth was removed. The abscess subsided. But the lymph node could still be felt although it was no longer tender. The family then went away for a holiday but Camilla was not quite well and the swelling of the lymph node became larger.

On return home her doctor found an **ulcer in her mouth** at the site of the tooth extraction and a **lymph node abscess**. The abscess was incised but did not heal. The skin around the incision was red and unhealthy. Two weeks later, and 6 weeks after the removal of the tooth TB were found in the discharge from the abscess.

Two weeks later Camilla awoke unusually early and **vomited**. The next day she was rather irritable and vomited again. She then complained of **headache** and it was obvious she was **losing weight**. On the seventh day of that episode she was sent to hospital with the clinical diagnosis of early **tuberculous meningitis**.

On **examination** she was thin, rather quiet and anxious, but quite alert and responsive. Both **neck and back stiffness** were found. In the left submandibular area there was an **ulcer** with a granulating base and thin undermined edges. The adjacent **lymph nodes** were firm and discrete. At the site of the tooth extraction there was a painless **ulcer** about 2.5 cm in diameter. In the mucous membrane surrounding the ulcer there were several small, 1 mm **yellow grey nodules**. The **spleen** was palpable but no other abnormal physical signs were found.

Lumbar puncture showed a cloudy fluid with 300 lymphocytes per mm^3 and 160 mg protein per cent. Soon the **tuberculin** reaction became positive.

Treatment was started and Camilla immediately began to improve. The signs of meningitis subsided. Within 2 weeks the ulcer in the mouth began to heal. Clinical recovery was complete. Later X-ray showed calcification at the site of the mandibular abscess.

Tuberculous meningitis following another infection and failure to take preventive chemotherapy

Dewi was the second of 3 sisters, one 2 years older and the other 2 years younger than herself. She was 4½ years old when the **whole family**, including her parents, had an **acute infective** illness with both cough and loose stools. She was the only one who did not recover quickly. She remained **vaguely ill**, **irritable** and had **occasional vomits** for about a week. She was then brought to hospital. On questioning the doctor found that about a year before her father had been discovered to have **chronic pulmonary tuberculosis** and had been treated. The children had all been examined. They had been found to be **tuberculin positive**. Their **X-rays** showed that Dewi and her elder sister each had a primary complex in the lung. At that time the children appeared to be in good health but, because of the tuberculin test and the X-ray findings, they were given chemotherapy. The parents did not accept this well. Treatment was only irregular and ceased entirely after about 3 months.

On **examination** at the hospital Dewi had a **headache**, her **words were slurred** and her **neck was stiff**. No choroidal tubercles were seen. On **lumbar puncture** the CSF was cloudy with 170 mg protein per cent and 960 cells per mm³. **TB** were seen on direct film and later cultured.

Dewi had been previously treated with isoniazid and ethambutol but both of these had been given together. So the doctor presumed the organisms were still sensitive. She was treated with isoniazid, rifampicin and pyrazinamide and made a rapid recovery.

3.5.2 Tuberculoma. Tuberculous deposits in the brain may become larger without rupturing or causing meningitis. The signs they cause depend where they are in the brain and the tracts they involve. As they increase in size they have the same effect as a brain tumour. The onset of symptoms and signs is usually slow. Any cranial nerve may be involved or the child may slowly develop a hemiplegia. In countries where tuberculosis is common any child who presents with the slow onset of signs of a cerebral tumour should be given a trial of anti-tuberculosis treatment.

3.5.3 Tuberculous arachnoiditis and paraplegia. Tuberculosis may attack the covering membrane of the spinal cord. This may be either an extension of a meningitis or a separate patch of inflammation. The nerves entering or leaving the spinal cord can be caught up in the process. The spinal cord itself can be compressed leading to stiffness or paralysis of the legs (paraplegia). The same symptoms may be due to tuberculous disease of **vertebrae** with the formation of an abscess which can compress the cord. You can easily recognise this if you can obtain an X-ray of the spine. But there may also be clinical evidence of disease in the vertebrae by the presence of an angular deformity of the spine produced by the collapse of the bodies of the vertebrae (Figure 21 p 64).

There is also another type in which the child has a raised temperature, stiffness of the neck and back and sometimes pains around the body or tenderness of the skin. If possible send the child to hospital for full investigation. If not possible, try the effect of anti-tuberculosis treatment and watch the result very carefully.

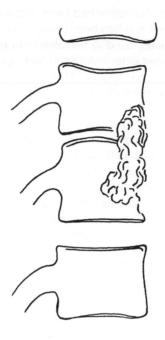

Figure 20   *Tuberculosis of spine:* diagram of X-ray. Note destruction of adjacent vertebrae and loss of disc space

3.6   Tuberculosis of bones and joints

TB can spread from the primary complex to any bone or joint. The risk that this will happen is greater the younger the child. Most bone or joint disease occurs within 3 years of the first infection but may be very much later. Although any bone or joint may be involved, those which are weight bearing are more likely to be affected than others. The spine is most frequently affected, then the hip, the knee and the bones of the foot; the bones of the arm or hand less often. Swellings in joints come on slowly without the heat and acute pain of a septic infection (though the joint is often a little warmer, when you lay your hand on it, than the unaffected joint in the other limb). The slow onset of a swelling either over a bone or a joint should make you think of tuberculosis.

As the clinical pictures are similar in adults and children these will be dealt with together in this section.

3.6.1 Tuberculosis of the spine
How it arises.   This arises from blood spread of TB. In about 70 per cent of patients two vertebral bodies are affected: in 20 per cent three or more.

It begins in the **anterior superior** (upper front) or **inferior** (lower) **angle** of the *body* and spreads to an adjacent (next) vertebra. The **disc** becomes involved and the disc space becomes narrowed (Figure 20). As the disease progresses an **abscess** forms and this may track to sites such as the lower thoracic cage or below the inguinal (groin) ligament (**psoas abscess**). It may also compress the spinal cord. The commonest site is T10. Frequency decreases the further the vertebra is from T10, above or below.

How it shows in the patient.   Tuberculous disease of the spine is not seen in the first year of life. It begins to appear after the child has learnt to walk and jump. After that it may occur at any age.

1. The first symptom is **pain**. To reduce this the child or adult holds his back stiffly. He refuses to bend to pick anything from the floor. If asked to do so he may bend at the knees keeping his back straight. The pain gets better if he rests.
2. **Signs at different levels**.
    a) In the **neck**. If the cervical vertebrae are involved the patient may not like to turn his head, and may sit with his chin propped up by his hand. He may feel pain in his neck or his shoulders. If an abscess tracks, a soft fluctuant swelling may appear on either side of the neck behind the sternomastoid muscle or bulge into the back of the mouth (pharynx).
    b) In the **back** down to the last rib (**thoracic region**). With disease in that region the patient has a stiff back. In turning he moves his feet rather than swings from the hips. When picking anything from the floor he bends his knees while his back remains stiff. Later there may be a visible lump or bend in the spine (**gibbus**) showing where the vertebral bodies have collapsed (Figure 21).
    c) If the **abscess** tracks it may pass to the right or the left round the chest and appear as a soft swelling on the chest wall. (A similar cold abscess can be due to tuberculosis of intercostal lymph nodes.) If it presses to the back it can compress the spinal cord and cause paralysis (**paraplegia** p 64 and 65).
    d) When the spine is affected lower than the chest (**lumbar region**) it is also below the spinal cord but the pus can track in muscles just as it did at higher levels. If that happens it may appear as a soft swelling either above or below the ligament in the groin or lower still on the inside of the thigh ('**psoas abscess**'). Rarely the pus can track through the opening in the pelvis and reach the surface behind the hip joint.
    (In high prevalence countries 1 in 4 patients with spinal tuberculosis has a clinically palpable abscess.)
3. In **malnourished** patients there may be fever (sometimes high fever), loss of weight and loss of appetite. In some Africans there may also

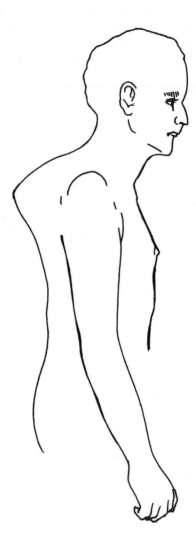

Figure 21   *Tuberculosis of spine: 'gibbus'*. Appearance of hump or lump in spine due to collapse of vertebral bodies

be enlarged **lymph nodes**, subcutaneous tubercles, enlargement of the **liver** and **spleen**.
4.   In **advanced disease** there may be not only a **gibbus** (angulation of the spine). There may also be weakness of the lower limbs and **paralysis** (paraplegia) due to pressure on the spinal cord or its blood vessels.

Investigations

1. If possible get antero-posterior and lateral X-rays. The common early features are loss of anterior superior or inferior angle of the body and loss of disc space (Figure 20). Remember that multiple lesions may be present in about 10 per cent of patients. A local abscess erodes the anterior surface of the bodies. An intrathoracic abscess may give rise to an appearance resembling an aortic aneurysm.

(2. **Blood tests** for anti-staphylococcal and anti-streptolysin haemolysins, typhoid, paratyphoid and brucellosis titres may help in difficult cases and in well-equipped centres.)

(3. **Needle biopsy** may also be useful in difficult cases but needs experience and good histology.)

4. Do not attempt to open an abscess. It will subside with treatment.

Complications. The main complication is weakness or paralysis of the legs. Loss of power is sometimes very rapid. If treated quickly it often responds well (in contrast to paralysis due to tumour etc.).

Differential diagnosis. In most cases the diagnosis is straightforward but tuberculosis may be confused with:

* **pyogenic infections** (e.g. staphylococcal)
* **enteric infections** (e.g. typhoid, paratyphoid)
* **tumours**

The X-ray appearances are usually characteristic. Evidence of new bone formation (sclerosis) would suggest pyogenic infection. Preservation of disc would suggest a tumour.

Treatment. This is discussed in detail on p 174.

AN ADULT PATIENT WITH SPINAL TUBERCULOSIS COMPLICATED BY PARAPLEGIA

Mrs Fraga, a 48-year-old woman complained of backache for several weeks. She went to her family doctor who told her that she had lumbago and told her to rest and apply local heat. The pain improved for a week or two, but became worse and began to keep her awake. Her family doctor sent her to hospital where she was X-rayed. The **X-ray** of spine was reported to show disease in the 9th and 10th thoracic vertebrae and that the diagnosis was malignant tumour. Because primary tumour of the spine is rare, her **chest was X-rayed** and showed almost **complete collapse of the left lower lobe**. The diagnosis then became primary tumour of the bronchus with secondary tumour in the spine. Radiotherapy was recommended. The following day she developed strange feelings in the legs and began to lose power in them (**paraplegia**).

The same day a physician who **specialised in tuberculosis** saw her. He pointed out that the X-ray of the spine showed **partial collapse of the vertebrae and loss of joint space** and that this was much more likely to be caused by tuberculosis. He recommended that she be examined by **bronchoscope**. She was found to have a large piece of **tuberculous tissue** from a **lymph node** obstructing the left lower lobe bronchus.

The physician immediately began chemotherapy and Mrs Fraga made a full recovery.

Comment. Remember that tuberculosis affects all age-groups – even those in whom cancer is more common. If there are facilities for investigation, use them to arrive at the right diagnosis: don't jump to conclusions. If diagnosed early, treatment of paraplegia (leg paralysis) due to tuberculosis of the spine is usually very successful – but not if the paralysis is due to tumour.

3.6.2 The hip. This is the second commonest place for bone tuberculosis. It is more common after than before 5 years of age. Young children may just become miserable, stop walking and refuse to walk if asked.

Older children and adults may **limp** and may complain of **pain** which sometimes is referred to the knee. The limp is due both to pain and to muscle spasm. If the condition is not recognised and treated the joint may be destroyed and the leg shortened.

If possible watch the child while he is playing or moving about so that any limp can be seen. Then examine him as he lies on his back at rest on a flat bench or table or even on the floor. It may not be easy to get him to do this if he is afraid or very young and patience is required. But if he will lie with his legs extended, gentle **rolling of each leg** will detect any spasm in the affected side. You must make sure that he is lying flat and not with his lumbar region arched forward. Slip your hand under his back to make sure. Any arching hides forward flexion of the hip. If the condition is advanced there may be shortening on the affected side. The thigh muscles are usually wasted (smaller). With a tape measure (or piece of string) compare the circumference with the normal side.

If possible **X-ray** films should be taken of both hips. Most disease begins inside the joint capsule but occasionally the joint appears clear and the disease is in the neck of the femur. First there is narrowing of the joint space between the acetabulum and the head of the femur but later there are changes in bone as the disease extends. In advanced cases the joint may be destroyed and the femur dislocated.

The slow onset, the results of the examination, the tuberculin test, and the X-ray if that is available should be sufficient to make the diagnosis and to start **treatment**. At the beginning the child should be at rest until the spasm disappears. The younger the child the greater the amount of bone regeneration that can be expected but in all children persistence with anti-tuberculosis treatment will bring a great measure of healing.

The history is sufficient to separate tuberculous arthritis from the acute, toxic and painful septic arthritis.

3.6.3. The knee joint. Disease in this joint usually begins slowly with swelling followed by pain. Indeed swelling may be the only sign. The swelling is due to fluid in the joint. The joint is often a little warmer than the opposite unaffected joint. Sometimes there is less fluid but thickened synovium (covering of the joint) may be felt above the patella (kneecap). Compare it with the opposite side. The thigh muscles are usually wasted (smaller). In these cases even if an X-ray is taken no bone changes may be found.

In other cases the first evidence of infection may be in the lower part of the femur or the upper part of the tibia and the changes in the joint are secondary to those in the bone.

A PATIENT WITH TUBERCULOSIS OF THE HIP FOLLOWING A FALL

Kadi aged 9 returned home one day and said he had **fallen** on his right leg. There was no obvious injury and next day he appeared well. About **a month later** he began to **drag that leg** and complained of **pain in the groin**. This limited his movement and he walked with a **limp**.

On **examination** there was some **wasting** of the right thigh. All **movements** of the right hip were **restricted**, particularly abduction (outward movement). Kadi's **elder sister** had had pulmonary tuberculosis for two years. His **tuberculin test** was strongly positive. **Chest X-ray** showed a healing primary lesion in the right lung. **X-ray of the right hip** showed narrowing of the joint space and some erosion of the acetabulum.

He was put on **bed rest** and began **chemotherapy**. Within a few days there was less muscle spasm. After 2 weeks joint movement was almost normal. He went on to make a complete recovery.

3.6.4 Ankle and small bones of the foot. As in other weight bearing joints pain and limp are early signs. Swelling over the affected bone or joint indicates the formation of an abscess. The calf muscles are often wasted (smaller). More than one lesion can be present and the same bones may be affected on each side. As in most tuberculosis of bone the swelling responds well to treatment. If the skin over the swollen area becomes red and fluctuant draw off the pus with a syringe. This may prevent a discharging sinus.

3.6.5 Arm and hand.   The upper limbs are less likely to be affected than the lower. Pain is less likely to be a complaint – again because weight bearing is less.

In the shoulder, elbow and wrist there is first some limitation of movement and then swelling about the joint. When the small bones of the **wrist** or the **fingers** are affected the lesions may be in the same bones on each side. Tuberculosis of the fingers (**dactylitis**) may show as an extended, somewhat oval, swelling of the finger, with less swelling round the proximal and terminal phalanges. Several fingers may be affected in each hand. (Infants with sickle cell anaemia may develop dactylitis but this is much more painful.)

As with other large joints, disease in the **shoulder** can begin either with an effusion into the joint or a bone focus in the head of the humerus; as movement is limited the muscles of the shoulder girdle become soft and wasted. Tuberculosis of the **elbow** joint follows the same pattern, reduction in movement, swelling of the joint. Since pain is so much less than in tuberculosis of the bones of the leg the child may not be seen until there is considerable destruction of the bone.

The first sign of tuberculosis infection of the **wrist** is nearly always a painless swelling over the back of the hand.

A PATIENT WITH TUBERCULOSIS OF THE ELBOW JOINT

Lamek was first seen when he was 2½ years old. Until he was aged 6 months he had been in frequent contact with an **aunt** who then **died of pulmonary tuberculosis**. He seemed to remain well for 2 years. Then his **left elbow joint** became stiff and movement was limited.

On **examination** he did not appear generally ill. The **left elbow joint** was swollen and all movements except pronation were limited. **Chest X-ray** showed many **calcified lymph nodes** at the hilum of the right lung. **X-ray of the elbow joint** showed gross bone destruction in the lower part of the humerus and upper ulna. There was marked loss of the joint surface of the ulna.

The doctor immobilised the elbow in a sling and started chemotherapy. He soon improved. Within 18 months there was good restoration of bone outline. The range of movement steadily increased as the joint was used. Finally he had practically full range of movement.

3.6.6 Other bones.   Although the bones of the spine and limbs are most affected, tuberculosis may appear in any bone. It usually shows as a painless swelling. This can slowly become red and discharge leaving a sinus. More than one swelling may be present.

Occasionally **multiple bone abscesses** may be seen, usually accompanied by fever. Though most are painless we have seen painful and tender abscesses in adults, though with little redness of the skin.

X-ray films will show the loss of bone shadowing at the site of the swelling.

3.6.7 *Cystic tuberculosis of bone.* This unusual type of bone tuberculosis needs special attention because it is so different from the sort just described. It is found in areas where tuberculosis is common and has been reported frequently from Africa. It appears as the slow growth of one or more hard painless swellings which do **not** affect the overlying skin to discharge or form abscesses. This appearance is most often found in the hands or feet. But it can also appear over the skull or in long bones particularly in the head of the humerus near the shoulder joint or in the head of the tibia. X-ray shows the swelling has cyst-like spaces with their walls giving a web-like appearance. These cysts are filled with caseation and contain large numbers of TB. Full treatment is required.

3.7 Tuberculosis of the eye

Tuberculosis affects the eyes more often than is realised. Bacilli can be lodged in the eye under the eyelids by dust or by the coughing of an infected person. Or they can reach the eye through blood spread from a primary focus or elsewhere.

There is also a painful condition – phlyctenular conjunctivitis – which is not due to direct infection but is probably a result of the 'sensitivity' to tuberculin which is being produced at the site of a primary focus in the chest or other site.

3.7.1 *Primary infection of the eye (conjuctiva).* If tubercle bacilli lodge under the upper or lower eyelid of a child who has not so far had a primary infection in the lung or abdomen they can multiply and form a tuberculous lesion. This is the same as a primary infection anywhere else. Multiplication is followed by caseation. You will find small yellow areas if you evert the eyelid.

This reaction does not cause the child much pain or difficulty. The eye may water and be rather irritable, the lid may become rather swollen. But as the process in the eye develops the lymph drainage from the area passes to the small lymph node just in front of the ear. This becomes involved in the tuberculous process, enlarges and may soften. It may be the swelling or softening, or even the rupture of the nodal abscess, which brings the child to seek help.

It is a good example of the fact that the first infection with tuberculosis always has both a place of entry of the bacilli and enlargement of the nearest lymph node.

From this type of infection bacilli can also escape into the bloodstream and be carried to other tissues such as bones just as they can from a primary infection in the lung. The treatment is the same as for primary infection in any site (p 76).

3.7.2 *Phlyctenular conjunctivitis.*

This painful reaction can occur at any time in tuberculous infection, but is commonest in the first year after infection. It begins with pain, irritation, lachrymation (tears) and photophobia (unwillingness to face light) in one or both eyes. One or more small grey or yellow spots are found round the limbus where the cornea meets the white of the eye. A number of small blood vessels run up from the edge of the conjunctival sac to meet the spots. Each spot lasts about a week and then slowly disappears. But it may be replaced by others.

In severe attacks the cornea may become ulcerated. Then pain is severe and the patient cannot bear light, either shading or closing his eyes or sitting in a dark corner.

If secondary infection should follow, there may be a purulent discharge and the cornea may be permanently scarred with white spots where the ulcers had formed.

This painful and sometimes repeated condition is most likely to occur between the ages of 5 and 15 years and is common in Africa, India and South-east Asia. It is usually due to tuberculosis, but can occur with infection by haemolytic streptococci.

Treatment.   The pupil should be kept dilated with 0.25 per cent atropine ointment: if there is no sign of secondary infection 1 per cent hydrocortisone drops will quickly bring relief but this cannot be used if infection is present or there is corneal ulceration. Continue the treatment of the primary infection.

3.7.3 *Choroidal (retinal) tubercles* (Figure 22).

Search of the retina with an ophthalmoscope after the pupil has been dilated with 0.25 per cent atropine ointment may sometimes establish the diagnosis of tuberculosis.

The examination is particularly worth doing when rapid diagnosis is required in cases of miliary spread (p 52 and 107) or tuberculous meningitis (p 58). As noted on p 58, in an ill, irritable child, it may be only possible to examine the retina thoroughly if the child is anaesthetised. This is well worth while in a difficult case.

As you look into the eye note the optic disc and the central artery of the retina which spreads out from its centre. Try to follow each of the main branches in turn as they spread into the retina. If tubercles are present and recent they appear as 1–3 mm yellowish, rounded, slightly raised spots. The edges fade into the general pinkness of the retina. They are most likely to be found within two disc-diameters of the centre of the optic disc. As the tubercle gets older the edge becomes more definite and the centre white.

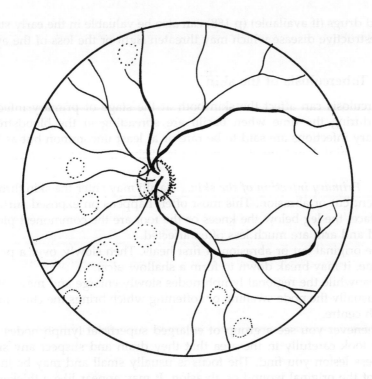

Figure 22   *Choroidal (retinal) tubercles*

If treatment begins when the tubercle is still yellow it can disappear entirely without leaving any scar but if it is white with a sharp edge when first seen that does not happen and the white area may slowly become filled with black pigmented dots.

3.7.4 *Acute tuberculous panophthalmitis.* This is a highly destructive abscess of the whole eye. The patient loses vision progressively and the whole of the eye becomes cloudy. Removal of the eye may be necessary eventually.

3.7.5 *Uveitis.* 'Mutton fat' lesions may occur on the back of the cornea and iris.

3.7.6 *Retinitis.* Greyish white ground glass blotches appear on the retina and the veins may be swollen with local haemorrhages.

Treatment of tuberculosis of the eye. All the above respond well to treatment with chemotherapy (children: p 76; adults: p 165). Corticos-

teroid drugs (if available) (p 188) can also be valuable in the early stages
of destructive disease which may threaten sight or the loss of the eye.

3.8 Tuberculosis of the skin

Tuberculosis can affect the skin both at the stage of primary infection
and during the time when bacilli are spreading in the bloodstream.
Primary infections are said to be rare or at least uncommon but as they
are not painful and are often small it is likely that many are missed.

3.8.1 Primary infection of the skin. Bacilli may enter the skin through
a recent cut or abrasion. This most often happens on exposed surfaces.
The face, the leg below the knees or the foot are the commonest places.
Hand and arm are much less often affected.

The original cut or abrasion at first heals. Then slowly, over a period
of time, it may break down to form a shallow ulcer.

Meanwhile the regional lymph nodes slowly enlarge and may soften.
It is usually the node swelling or softening which brings the child to the
health centre.

Whenever you see a group of enlarged superficial lymph nodes you
must look carefully in the area that they drain and suspect any small
painless lesion you find. The focus is usually small and may be in the
scar of the original wound or abrasion. It may appear like a thickening
of the skin and be surrounded by tiny yellowish spots also set in the
skin. If the infection has been there for some months before the regional
nodes have softened the focus may have healed to give a central area of
smooth scar with a sharply defined irregular edge. The tiny yellow areas
will have left sharply defined little pits.

A similar appearance may sometimes be seen in the scar at the site of
a BCG infection for this also produces a primary skin infection.

3.8.2 Abscesses. Two types of tuberculous abscess occur in addition to
those which might come from lymph nodes or bones.

1. The first appears as a soft swelling just under the skin. More than
   one may be present in different parts of the body at the same time.
   Being just under the skin they soon rupture to form an ulcer which
   usually has a very irregular edge and a clean base. If the child's
   nutrition is good the ulcers slowly heal. But remember that the child
   may have other tuberculous lesions.
2. The other type of abscess can follow an **intra-muscular injection**. It
   is deeper and larger than those described above. Since they follow
   an injection they are found in injection sites, mostly on the buttocks
   but sometimes on the outside of the thigh or arm. If the infection
   results from a dirty needle and the child has not previously had a

primary infection then the regional lymph nodes are also enlarged and the child may develop tuberculosis in other organs.

3.8.3 *Single large painless skin lesions.* These are sometimes seen on the hand or face. They are set deeply in the skin. Small at first they can reach 2.5–5 cm and become covered with scaly rough skin. Usually they remain unchanged for months before slowly healing to leave a scar through the thickness of the skin.

3.8.4 *Erythema nodosum and other types of tuberculous skin disease.* These are covered in the adult section (p 131).

3.9 Unusual places for children's tuberculosis

3.9.1. *The genital tract*

Primary infection. In areas or countries where **male circumcision** is done as a matter of custom infection of the wound with tubercle bacilli has often been recorded. When this happens the wound may at first heal and then break down to form the primary focus. The lymph from it drains to the nodes in the groin – usually both sides. These then enlarge and may form abscesses.

Any circumcision wound which does not heal and is followed by enlargement of the nodes on one or both sides should therefore raise the suspicion of tuberculosis.

When the operation is carried out in infants the risk of blood spread and the development of miliary disease or meningitis is high.

Similar risks must arise following **female circumcision** when again a local lesion and node swellings would develop though the risk of blood spread would vary with the age of the child (p 43).

Blood spread disease. In **boys** before puberty the epididymis just above the testis may become swollen and at first hard. The lump may later soften and discharge through the skin. In young children it is usually only one of a number of lesions in a blood spread disease. In older boys the testis alone or both testis and epididymis are more likely to be affected; both enlarge and become attached to the skin and if not treated can soften and discharge.

The process is slow, chronic and relatively painless: it is quite different from an acute bacterial infection with fever, pain, swelling and tenderness of the testis. This is usually part of a urinary infection.

In young **girls** tubercles can occur in the **uterus** and **fallopian tubes** as part of the blood spread after primary infection in the lung. These organs can also be involved in tuberculosis of the **abdominal cavity** following the rupture of a mesenteric node after a primary infection of the intestinal tract.

But pelvic tuberculosis with disease in the uterus or the fallopian tubes is most usually caused by blood spread from a pulmonary primary infection which has occurred after puberty when the blood supply to the pelvic organs is so much increased. This is important because even if it does not cause symptoms of local disease at the time it can cause infertility in later years. For this reason many doctors would give chemoprophylaxis with isoniazid (p 197) to tuberculin positive girls without symptoms.

Primary tuberculosis in adolescent girls should always be treated.

If disease does develop the **symptoms** are lower abdominal pain, loss of weight or appetite, sometimes with lower abdominal distension and amenorrhoea.

On **examination** a mass may be felt in the pelvis either centrally or to one or the other side. There may be signs of tuberculosis elsewhere in the body. If possible get an X-ray of the chest. The response to treatment is usually good and it should be started as soon as possible.

For details of disease in adults see p 126.

3.9.2 The kidneys.   Tuberculosis of the urinary system is not often seen in children because it only develops 7–10 years after the primary infection (Figure 17, p 42).

The infection reaches the kidney by the bloodstream. It develops slowly, beginning between the pyramid and the cortex of the kidney and causing caseation just as it does in the lung.

Usually the slow extension opens into the pelvis of the kidney and caseous material is carried in the urine down to the bladder which may also become diseased.

The **symptoms** of disease may be slight unless the bladder is involved when there is frequent passing of urine and sometimes pain. If there is apparent cystitis, with pus in the urine, but the urine is sterile on culture, remember the possibility of tuberculosis.

When blood is passed in the urine without a complaint of pain tuberculosis should always be considered and the patient sent where investigation is possible. Of course blood in the urine is very common in areas where there is bilharzia. But remember the possibility of tuberculosis. The treatment of all primary infections so that blood spread of bacilli is made harmless would greatly reduce the incidence of renal tuberculosis or rule it out completely.

Genito-urinary disease in adults is covered in more detail on p 123.

3.9.3. The liver and spleen.   After primary infection, when bacilli are spreading, both the liver and the spleen may become enlarged. This is most marked in young children when the blood spread is heavy (miliary tuberculosis p 51). But there are many other causes of enlarged liver and spleen. Always consider the whole clinical picture.

Primary infection can occur in the liver of a fetus infected from the mother (section 3.10 below).

3.9.4 Tuberculous pericarditis.   See p 118.

3.10   Infection before (congenital) or during birth or in the newborn period

If tubercle bacilli pass through the placenta from the mother's circulation to the fetal circulation, infection can occur. Babies can also be infected during or immediately after birth by the inhalation of infected material, or from a birth attendant or other person who has active pulmonary tuberculosis and positive sputum. If a child was infected before birth, the mother must have had tuberculosis during pregnancy. The TB must have reached the fetus through the mother's blood. The mother must have either had a recent primary infection or progressive disease. During a recent primary infection there is often a period when bacilli pass into the bloodstream.

The bacilli pass through the placenta and enter the fetal circulation. Next the bacilli are carried by the umbilical veins to the liver. Most of the infants seem well at birth but by about the third week the baby stops gaining **weight** and becomes **jaundiced**, with **pale stools and dark urine**. The liver and spleen are found to be enlarged. The infant has obstructive jaundice because there is a primary focus in the liver and large lymph nodes obstruct the outflow of bile at the porta hepatis. The other causes of jaundice at this period should be excluded.

Sometimes organisms pass through the ductus venosus to the heart and lungs which are the site of infection. If the child has been infected during or immediately after birth the illness does not become apparent for 3–4 weeks and then quickly resembles an acute **pneumonia**. The first signs may be attacks of cyanosis or a cough, but the illness increases rapidly and fine moist sounds can be heard on both sides of the chest. If an X-ray is taken there are inflammatory changes on both sides, often thought to be an acute pneumonia. The only hope is to consider the possibility of tuberculosis and examine the stomach washings. TB are usually very numerous. The tuberculin test is negative. As soon as diagnosis is made full treatment must be given (p 76). A number of children have recovered.

See also p 165 for guidance on the care of the newborn child of a mother with tuberculosis. Of course you should treat any pregnant mother who has tuberculosis, both for her own sake and for the baby's sake. Avoid streptomycin which can cause deafness in the infant.

4: HOW YOU CAN HELP AND TREAT TUBERCULOUS CHILDREN

When the child's history, symptoms and physical signs and score according to Score Chart A (Table 3 p 48) suggest that he has tuberculosis you must make a series of decisions.

1. If a National Tuberculosis Programme is in operation and the policy is laid down for you, then you should comply with it. See that your patient comes under the care of that programme as soon as possible. Local conditions vary and they will of course affect your decisions.
2. If you yourself must initiate and supervise the child's care and treatment it will help you to think of four needs:
    a) the drugs (chemotherapy) required for tuberculosis
    b) medicine required for other infections or infestations
    c) attention to the child's nutrition
    d) protection against infections which reduce resistance to tuberculosis, particularly measles and whooping cough.

You should consider separately each of these aspects of help.

4.1 Anti-tuberculosis medicines

When you suspect a child has tuberculosis the immediate action you will have to take will depend on the situation in which you are working. There are many variations but they can be summarised into these major categories.

1. When you are able to transport or send the child and his/her family to a larger hospital or tuberculosis centre where he/she may be investigated further and if necessary treated. If you send children and their families to other centres find out later what happens to them.
2. When the child is so ill that although you can send him to a larger centre you consider that treatment should be started immediately. This would apply to children with extensive pulmonary involvement, with meningitis or miliary tuberculosis. In this situation you will have made your assessment according to the Score Chart A (p 48). Initially if the score has been 6 or less and there were signs of 'pneumonia' you would have treated with a broad spectrum antibiotic according to the Flow Chart B. But if there is no improvement you should start anti-tuberculosis chemotherapy. You would send full clinical notes with the child.
3. When you must treat the child yourself, if possible follow the course prescribed for children in your National Tuberculosis Programme.

Also pay attention to the important aspects of care which are described later in this section.

If there is not a schedule of treatment laid down in a National Programme you might be limited by the supply of drugs you have available or can obtain.

The following approach is, however, flexible and will allow you to do your best whatever your circumstances.

Children who require drug treatment fall into several clinical groups.

1. Children of all ages **without symptoms of illness** who are known to have had a recent primary tuberculosis infection. The object is to remove the risk of disseminated lesions and to kill the TB in the primary focus and regional nodes of the complex. The treatment should rely upon isoniazid (INH) 5 mg/kg given once daily for a minimum of 6 months.

   You may find other children without evidence of disease but with a strongly positive tuberculin reaction. You may not know when they developed the primary infection. Because of the risk of blood spread in young children (under age 5) most agree that these should be treated with INH alone (as above). The risk is lower at older ages and what you do should depend on recommendations of your National Programme, your local facilities (e.g. drug supplies) and the circumstances of the particular child.

2. Children **with symptoms** who have **pulmonary or non-pulmonary disease**, such as bone or joint tuberculosis.

   a) Treat according to your National Programme.

   b) If there is no guidance from this, or no programme, use IUATLD/WHO recommended treatment. Give a 6-month regimen with INH and rifampicin (RIF), together with pyrazinamide (PZA) for the first 2 months (doses given below). Give the drugs in a single dose a day, if possible before a meal.

   c) In several African countries the above regimen is given for the first 2 months only, followed by INH and thioacetazone (Tb1) in a single dose a day for 6 months (8 months treatment in all). If there are side-effects to Tb1 complete treatment with INH alone. (Some countries treat for 12 months using only Tb1 and INH throughout.)

3. Children who are **seriously ill** with extensive pulmonary disease, with miliary tuberculosis, or with tuberculous meningitis. Here the situation is urgent and you should start treatment at once. If there is no guidance from your National Programme, treat as in para 2b above. For further details of treatment for tuberculous meningitis see p 176).

   Watch the patient carefully for improvement. The first signs may be that the child becomes more aware, and better able to take food and drink. The temperature may begin to come down.

Table 4   *Doses of drugs for children*

	Daily	Intermittent
Isoniazid (INH)	5 mg/kg	15 mg/kg
(Tuberculous meningitis:	10 mg/kg)	
Rifampicin (RIF)	10 mg/kg	10 mg/kg
		(max 900 mg)
Pyrazinamide (PZA)	25 mg/kg	× 3/week:
		50 mg/kg
Thioacetazone (Tb1)	2.5 mg/kg	unsuitable

Important notes:
1. In the past many paediatricians have used a dose of 10 mg/kg of INH. IUATLD and WHO do **not** recommend this, except in the early stages of treating meningitis.
2. **We do not now recommend using streptomycin** for children. This is for three reasons: a) Streptomycin injections are painful. b) Unless there is very careful sterilisation of syringes there is a risk of spreading HIV. c) Providing syringes adds to the cost.
3. For thioacetazone treatment 1 standard tablet: 50 mg Tb1 + 100 mg INH. Because of dangerous side-effects some HIV high prevalence countries are ceasing to use Tb1.
4. For **side-effects** of drugs see p 186.

4.1.1 Other points in treatment.   You may meet a child with a primary infection who **does not appear to be ill** but you judge needs treatment with preventive INH (p 197). It is understandable that the parents may be unwilling to give the child 'medicine' when they cannot see that he is 'ill'. You must talk to them slowly and carefully, and give them clear answers to their questions. Can you find a parallel in nature where you do something to kill a pest on plants or in animals before they can do harm rather than waiting for the signs of disease? After all, prophylactic (preventive) medicine is only difficult to accept because they cannot see the thing you are treating. And of course they may not believe the germ theory of disease. (See also p 16.)

When a child is being treated for tuberculosis he will often soon feel much better, put on weight, and become more active well before the treatment is finished. The parents may think that they can then stop the treatment. Explain that the purpose of the treatment is not only to stop the growth of and to kill the bacilli but to heal the damage they have done. The patient feels better when the medicine stops the bacilli growing. But then the medicine must be continued while the body slowly heals the area where the bacilli have been or allows bone to grow normally again.

Always use a weight chart to show weight change in relation to treatment.

4.2   Other medicines

When you treat a child for tuberculosis you must not forget that he may also have **other conditions** (infective or otherwise). These may need treatment. This, of course, will also help in the general recovery of his health.

In areas where **parasites** are frequent, you should examine the child for these and treat if necessary. Malaria is only one example.

Worm infections, ascariases, hookworm and tapeworms vary in their frequency from one place to another. You will know what is common in your district. Treat any infestation you find.

Children may also have evidence of **other infections**. The most common are those of the upper respiratory tract, with nasal discharge and obstruction and maybe discharge from one or both ears. If one or both ears are discharging you should, if possible, try to find out whether the discharge contains any TB. (See p 55.)

In your examination you may also find that the child has **ulcers** or **pustules** or **boils**. Protect these and treat locally. Also give an antibiotic effective against the commonest organisms, staphylococci and streptococci. Skin sores or ulcers may also become infected with diphtheria.

Anaemia, secondary to insufficient intake of iron or to blood loss, is common. You should check the child's haemoglobin as part of the first examination. Correct anaemia with tabs ferrous sulphate or tabs fersolate (200 mg ferrous sulphate). Dose: infants ½ tablet twice daily; 2–5 years, 1 tablet twice daily; school children 1 tablet three times a day.

Always treat attacks of **diarrhoea** promptly and with care. Teach parents oral rehydration and encourage feeding. They should use simple methods (spoon or cup). Make sure they know how to make sugar and salt solution or know how to use packets of oral rehydration salts (UNICEF and WHO). If possible dissolve them in clean water – boiled if necessary. But boiled water takes a long time to cool. If the child is desperately ill use the cleanest available water.

You should have a practical guide to the measurement of diarrhoea of different degrees of severity and duration. For this *Practical Care of Sick Children* by P. Dean and G.J. Ebrahim is a useful book. It is designed for use in small hospitals in tropical situations. (Published by Macmillans, a low cost edition for export to countries outside Europe, North America and Japan can be obtained through TALC, Box 49, St Albans, Herts AL1 4AX, UK.)

4.3   Food and nutrition

Tuberculosis and malnutrition travel hand in hand. Infection with tuberculosis causes loss of weight and wasting; insufficient food increases the risks of infection and then the spread of tuberculous disease. You must always think of nutrition and food with the same care and concern that you think of tuberculosis itself, and of the dangers of other infective illnesses. You must remember that they affect each other.

When you examine a child always look for signs of malnutrition. Weigh the child and enter the weight on the growth chart. Look at the child's behaviour. Does the child seem hungry or apathetic? Check the quality of hair and skin. Look for skin rash. Is there normal subcutaneous fat? Is there oedema of the feet?

From this you will form a first impression of the state of nutrition and whether the situation is urgent.

Decide whether to admit the child to hospital for special observation and treatment. This will include educating the parents, particularly in how to help with the urgent job of improving the child's nutrition. (The small book recommended in section 4.2 contains detailed guidance in this most important part of treatment.)

The child who is very ill and malnourished may be unwilling to take food. Offer small amounts of food often. Nasogastric drip may be necessary until some appetite returns. At first milk (cows', goats', dried or evaporated) can be used with added sugar (50 g or 10 teaspoonfuls to the litre). In severe cases give ½ strength feeds every 2 hours to reduce the risk of diarrhoea. Continue for about 3 days and then high energy milk feeds can be used. These are prepared by adding vegetable oils to the milk feed and are valuable because they provide extra energy (see Table 5, but also consult your books on the nursing and care of malnourished children).

An ill, malnourished child easily becomes hypothermic (low temperature). Hypothermia is very dangerous and further reduces the body's defences. Make sure the child is nursed in a warm place. Mother's warm skin is the best source of heat. Make cotton wool hat and bootees to cover head and feet.

In such children give a **multivitamin preparation** daily. Also give one dose by mouth of vitamin A 200,000 units in oil on one occasion to prevent eye complications. UNICEF distributes K-Mix 2 for the treatment of protein energy malnutrition – 100 g of K-Mix 2 and 50 g (58 ml) of vegetable oil to which add slowly 1 litre of water while stirring well.

When the child's appetite returns, begin to introduce the usual local foods to replace the high energy milk. The mother should always be involved in this care which, for her, will be useful education.

4.4   Immunisation and protection

It is well known that measles and whooping cough lower the resistance to tuberculosis. Spread of tuberculosis may occur after a child with a primary infection has had either of those common illnesses. Whenever

Table 5 *Preparation of special milk feeds* (Courtesy of Drs P. Dean and G.J. Ebrahim: Reference 12)

High energy milk feeds, preparation of 1 litre using tablespoon and cups (250 ml)

Methods of preparation

Base content	Milk (amount)	Oil (tablespoons)	Sugar (tablespoons)
Cows' or goats' milk	3¾ cups	5	7
Skimmed milk	13 tbsp	8	7
Full cream milk powder	15 tbsp	5	7
Evaporated milk	1¾ cups	5	6
K-Mix powder	10 tbsp	8	4

For treatment of protein calorie malnutrition

K-Mix 2

Prepared	Calcium caseinate	3 parts by weight
by	Skimmed milk powder	5 parts by weight
UNICEF	Sucrose	10 parts by weight
	Retinol palmitate	2.75 mg (5,000 IU Vitamin A per 100 mg dry mixture)

Control
When the child is improving and appetite has returned, you must continue to teach the need for plenty of suitable food and also make sure that the mother both understands that need and is able to prepare the food required.

Make sure also that the child is weighed regularly and the weight recorded on a chart (Road to Health Chart). Weight gain is the easiest and best objective sign of improvement.

you treat a child for any form of tuberculosis you should check on his or her clinical history and immunisation state.

If there is no reasonable evidence that the child has been immunised or has previously had measles or whooping cough, do all you can to see that he is brought into the WHO Expanded Program on Immunization scheme and protected.

You should be familiar with the immunisation policy that is followed in your area and should check as far as possible that all children under your care are protected. Record all immunisations which you give. Also record them on a card which the parents keep.

4.5 Always remember

Tuberculosis in children can easily be missed, and often is, but **you** will not miss it if you always keep it in your mind. Always remember the four questions set out at the beginning of this chapter (p 29).

In children you must think of tuberculosis as a general disease which may appear in any part of the body – not, as usually in adults, with cough and sputum which may be blood stained. The ways it does show itself are given in answer to question three (p 44).

In children it is difficult to prove the diagnosis by finding TB. This does not mean that you should not try (p 46) but it **does** mean that you must not delay treatment when your clinical judgement tells you that the tuberculosis is likely. This may be either because the illness fits into one of those described under question three (p 44) or because a chronic condition in the chest, lymph nodes, a bone or joint, in the abdomen or elsewhere has failed to respond to other treatments.

When you treat tuberculosis in a child, the child's condition and behaviour usually improve quickly. Listen carefully to what the mother says. She is often the first to notice a change. Train yourself to **look carefully at your patients as persons** as well as at the complaint or symptom which brought them to you. **Whoever they are, they need to feel you care for them.**

5: HIV INFECTION, AIDS (ACQUIRED IMMUNODEFICIENCY SYNDROME) AND TUBERCULOSIS IN CHILDREN*

HIV (human immunodeficiency virus) infection is now spreading rapidly in many countries, especially in Africa and SE Asia. Many women of reproductive age are infected and give birth to infected babies. Immune deficiency due to HIV is now responsible for many hospital admissions. It is a major cause of infant mortality in some countries.

5.1 Where infection comes from

The most common route of infection is from **mother to child** during pregnancy or at birth. The risk of an infected mother passing on HIV to her child is between 20 per cent and 40 per cent. The risk may be higher when the mother develops symptoms or clinical AIDS.

Blood transfusions are another important cause of infection when

---

*We are grateful to Dr Wendy Holmes, who has had considerable experience of HIV infection in African children, for the bulk of the following account.

blood cannot be screened for HIV antibodies. Even where blood is screened, there must be strict rules for transfusion when HIV infection is common in the population. This is because a donor who has been recently infected may give blood before antibodies develop.

Breastfeeding is not an important route of infection with HIV. It is true that HIV has been cultured from breast milk and there are several reports of HIV infection apparently through breastfeeding. But in most of these cases the mother was infected by blood transfused after delivery. The risk of infection from breast milk will be very small compared with the risk of infection during pregnancy. There are many reports of babies who were breastfed by their HIV infected mothers but who did not become infected. Breastfeeding has many advantages. Babies infected with HIV need the protection against infection that breast milk provides. So **encourage HIV infected mothers to breastfeed their babies**, unless the mother is very ill.

Contaminated syringes and needles are another possible route of infection.

5.2 Diagnosis

The HIV antibody test is unreliable in the early diagnosis of HIV infection in children. Because the mother's antibodies cross the placenta, almost all babies born to HIV positive mothers have HIV antibodies in their blood at birth. Most of the **uninfected** babies lose their maternal HIV antibodies by 15 months. Most **infected** babies go on to produce their own antibodies, so in them the antibody test remains positive after 15 months. But some babies known to be infected with HIV have a negative test for HIV antibodies. The reason for this is not known. So in babies under 15 months it is best to diagnose by clinical signs and symptoms in the baby and a positive HIV antibody test in the mother.

5.3 Age when children become ill

A few infected babies become ill in the first weeks of life. In some children symptoms and signs are delayed for years. But most children who develop symptoms of infection become ill before 2 years of age. Progress is usually more rapid in children than adults. We do not yet know what factors influence the age when actual AIDS disease develops. It is possible that tuberculosis allows the virus to multiply more quickly and so speeds the development of the AIDS illness.

5.4 Ways in which HIV infection shows in children

HIV infection in children may show in a wide variety of ways. This means that the disease is difficult to define clinically. The WHO clinical definition for AIDS illness in children is not very specific. It can be confused with other diseases. AIDS most commonly shows as fever, with cough, failure to thrive, chronic diarrhoea and itchy rash. Suspect HIV infection when the child has a combination of the signs and symptoms in the following list:

*Major criteria for WHO definition**
Weight loss or abnormally slow growth
Chronic diarrhoea for more than one month
Prolonged fever for more than one month
Minor criteria for WHO definition
Generalised enlargement of lymph nodes
Thrush (fungal infection) in mouth and throat
Recurrent common infections (e.g. ear infections, pharyngitis)
Persistent cough
Generalised rash
Other common manifestations
Neurological problems
Delay in development
Enlargement of parotid glands on both sides
Enlarged spleen
Enlarged liver
Recurrent abscesses
Meningitis
Herpes simplex

It is important to ask about the mother's and father's health. Examine the mother if possible. General enlargement of lymph nodes in the mother or scars of herpes zoster (shingles) can be a useful clue to the diagnosis.

5.5   Diagnosing it from other diseases

Tuberculosis, malnutrition and chronic diarrhoea cause the greatest problems. This is even more difficult because all three of these may also occur in HIV infected children. Several features are common to tuberculosis and HIV infection. These include failure to thrive, loss of weight, intermittent fever, chronic cough, enlargement of liver or spleen, and history of recurrent illnesses. General enlargement of lymph nodes is rarer with tuberculosis but more common in children with HIV. Chest X-ray appearances may be similar. Because of reduced immunity, the tuberculin test is often negative in a child who has both HIV infection and tuberculosis.

---

*WHO clinical case definition of AIDS in children: diagnose AIDS if there are two or more major criteria + two or more minor criteria (which include, in addition, confirmed HIV infection in the mother), without any other known cause of immune suppression.

5.6   Prognosis

The prognosis seems to vary with the age when AIDS develops. Many infected children stop growing and suffer frequent infections before they are 1 year old. They often deteriorate and then die in the second or third year of life. Other children develop symptoms for the first time in their second or third year. These children often continue to grow well despite frequent minor illnesses. If the child has poor nutrition as well as HIV he/she is very vulnerable to fatal infections. Some HIV infected children remain completely well. They may become ill years later, but we know little about this group because AIDS is a new disease.

5.7   Tuberculosis in HIV infected children

The natural history of tuberculosis in an HIV infected child depends on the stage of the HIV disease. If the HIV infection has not yet shown itself and the child still has good immunity, we can expect the same signs of tuberculosis as in an uninfected child. But TB are more likely to spread to other parts of the body in a child who has HIV infection. Tuberculous meningitis, miliary tuberculosis, and general enlargement of lymph nodes are all more likely to occur. With this difficulty in diagnosis, always consider the possibility of tuberculosis in an HIV infected child. When an HIV infected child loses weight for several months and develops recurrent infections or chronic cough, it is easy to assume that there is nothing more you can do for them. However a very ill HIV infected child may respond well to anti-tuberculosis chemotherapy. When symptoms are suggestive of tuberculosis it is always worth trying the effect of chemotherapy. You must watch the child carefully and weigh him/her frequently to decide whether there is a response to treatment.

If the child responds to treatment try to arrange for him to continue treatment at home. Avoid long hospital admissions. Hospital admissions expose these children with little immunity to many risks of infection. It also disrupts family life. Do not use streptomycin injections. These injections are painful and increase the risk of spreading HIV infection. Remember also that these children may have other treatable infections (see p 141).

5.8   Counselling

When you suspect that a child may be infected with HIV, it is important to counsel the mother and obtain her consent before you test her blood. When you tell a mother that you suspect her child might have HIV infection you give her a great deal of bad news. Her child may have an incurable and fatal disease. She may be infected herself. Her husband may be infected. Any future babies may also be infected.

Try to give her plenty of time to understand, and to ask questions. Discuss the possible advantages and disadvantages of a test for her. If she knows that she is HIV infected she will be able to make important decisions about the future. On the other hand, she may fear that her husband will leave her if she has a positive result. Always ask the mother whether she would like to bring her husband for counselling **before** she has the test. A woman will often find it easier to tell her husband about the possibility of HIV infection than to tell him afterwards that she has a positive result.

Parents also need counselling when the results are known. Advise them about the outlook for the child and the risk to future babies. Explain how HIV infection spreads. Encourage them to change any behaviour that may put other people at risk. Parents will need continued support and counselling to help them to come to terms with the bad news. Common reactions include shock, anger, guilt, grief and depression. It is helpful to train nurses or other health workers in HIV counselling so that they can give enough time to this important aspect of management. (See also p 142.)

5.9   HIV infection and BCG

There have been reports of disseminated BCG in children who have HIV related suppression of their immunity. In an uninfected child the immune system limits the BCG infection to the site of vaccination. But in immune suppressed children the bacilli are able to spread through the body.

WHO recommends that children with **symptoms of HIV disease** should not receive BCG. However, in countries with high prevalence of tuberculosis, **HIV infected children who are well** should still receive BCG vaccination. HIV infection is difficult to diagnose in the newborn. The newborn infant may be seropositive because it has received anti-bodies, but not virus, from its mother. So WHO recommends that well infants of HIV infected mothers **should** be given BCG.

If BCG dissemination does occur it can be successfully treated with rifampicin and isoniazid. As BCG originally came from a bovine strain it is resistant to pyrazinamide. But though the BCG dissemination may be controlled, unfortunately the infant is likely to die from its AIDS.

References

Harries A.D., Maher D. *TB/HIV. A Clinical Manual.* Geneva: WHO, 1997.

WHO Global Programme on AIDS. *Counselling for HIV/AIDS: a key to caring.* Geneva: WHO, 1995.

WHO Global Programme on AIDS. *AIDS In Africa. A Manual for Physicians.* Geneva: WHO, 1992.

3
Pulmonary Tuberculosis in Adults

1: LUNG TUBERCULOSIS IN ADULTS

1.1 How pulmonary tuberculosis develops in adults

On p 31 we described how lung lesions might arise from the primary lesion in a child. Here we describe what may happen in adults.

In an adult pulmonary tuberculosis may arise from:

1. **Progression of a primary lung infection** (Figure 23 a to d) in a person who has never previously been infected (previously tuberculin negative). In adults the primary lesion is often in the apex or the upper zone of the lung. In the adult primary complex, the lung lesion is often more obvious than the lymph node enlargement, which you may not be able to detect on an X-ray. Progression to the adult type of lung disease (worsening and spreading) of a new primary lesion is more likely after puberty than in the younger child. This is a common way for tuberculosis to develop in young adults.
2. Progression of lung lesions coming from the **blood spread** of bacilli, which normally occurs after a primary lesion (p 35). These bacilli may end up in the lung as in other organs (Figure 24, p 89). If there are many bacilli and defences are poor, miliary tuberculosis results. If there are only a few bacilli and good defences the bacilli may be killed. In between, lesions may start at one or both apices of the lung and later spread to other areas. This is an uncommon way for adult tuberculosis to develop.
3. **Reactivation of an earlier primary lesion**, perhaps years after a childhood infection by TB. The patient's defences may have kept the lesion under control in childhood, but lowering of the patient's defences (e.g. by malnutrition, pregnancy, parturition, other disease: p 11) may allow the TB to become active and spread the disease. This is a common way for tuberculosis to develop in middle or old age.
4. **Reactivation of an old postprimary lesion** which had been partially healed.

In adults of European origin, the **lymph node components** (hilar or

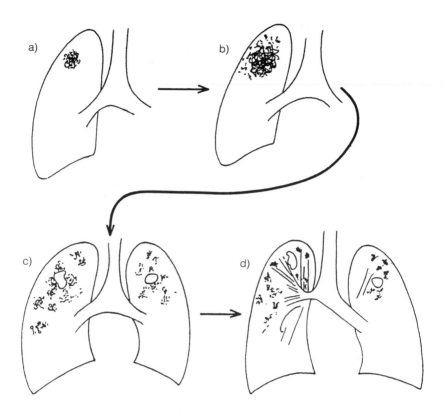

Figure 23   *X-ray appearances of progression (worsening) of primary lesion in an adult.*
a) Primary lung lesion in an adult. It is often in the upper part of the lung. The
lesion in the hilar lymph node is often not visible on the X-ray (though sometimes
– in Africans, Asians or patients with HIV infection – the nodes may be greatly
enlarged). The lung and lymph node lesions often heal and may later calcify. But
there may be: **b)** Gradual **enlargement of the lung lesion. c) Caseation** of the
lesion. Liquified caseous material may be coughed up. This results in a **cavity**.
Spread of TB from the cavity to produce further lesions in the same and in the
opposite lung (with a further cavity developing in that lung). **d)** After a year or
two (if the patient survives) development of **fibrosis** (scarring) which pulls up
the right hilum and pulls the trachea over to the right. **Calcification** is starting
in older apical lesions. Note the cavities are still open. This type of 'chronic
survivor' is a major source of infection.

paratracheal) of the primary complex are usually not visible in an X-ray.
But in Asians or Africans they may be very prominent; and the patient
sometimes has high fever. This is also seen in tuberculosis complicating
HIV infection. In these races and in patients with HIV, tuberculous

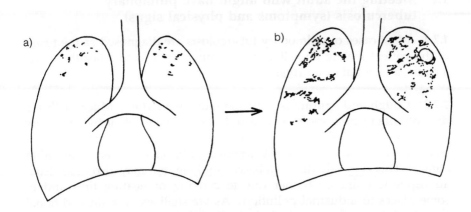

Figure 24 *X-ray appearance of blood spread origin of some types of pulmonary tuberculosis.* **a)** Blood spread of TB from the primary lesion (invisible) to form **small lesions at the apex of both lungs**. Higher oxygen in this part of the lungs encourages the growth of the bacilli. **b)** Lesions have become **confluent** (run together). A **cavity** has developed on the left. Disease has spread to the midzone of each lung

enlargement of hilar or paratracheal nodes may sometimes occur months or years after the primary infection.

In adults tuberculous lesions occur particularly in the **upper parts of the lungs** because, as mentioned in the caption to Figure 24, the oxygen level is higher there; this helps the TB to grow.

Spread within the lung often results from the caseation (cheesy necrosis) in the lesion, followed by breakdown into liquid material. The liquid material is coughed up, leaving an air-containing **cavity**. TB multiply rapidly in the cavity and can spread through the bronchi to new areas of lung. Lesions may be patchy, or they may join together to form **tuberculous pneumonia**. This may again break down into further cavities.

The lesions may heal by **fibrosis** or scar tissue. There can be a mixture with worsening in some areas and fibrosis occurring at the same time in others. Some lesions may **calcify**, showing as white material on the X-ray. Later the fibrosis may shrink so that, on the X-ray, the hilar shadows may be pulled up or the trachea be pulled over to that side. The lesions may damage the walls of the bronchi and produce **bronchiectasis**, with gross widening of the bronchi. As the bronchiectasis is usually in the upper lobes and is well drained by gravity mostly it does not cause symptoms itself (apart from the symptoms of tuberculosis).

1.2 Meeting the adult who might have pulmonary tuberculosis (symptoms and physical signs)

1.2.1 Most cases of pulmonary tuberculosis are diagnosed as the result of the patient feeling unwell and so coming for help to a health centre, a clinic, a hospital or a private doctor.

1.2.2 **Cough and sputum** is very common everywhere. Much of this is due to acute respiratory infections and lasts only a week or two. In many countries there is also much chronic cough due to chronic bronchitis (sometimes called 'Chronic Obstructive Pulmonary Disease' or other names). This is mostly due to tobacco smoking, but may also occur from atmospheric pollution (either due to cooking or heating fires and in some places to industrial pollution). As we shall see, certain additional symptoms may suggest tuberculosis. But often this is not obvious: **the only way to make sure is to examine the sputum for TB in everyone who has had a cough for more than 3 weeks.**

1.2.3 Here follow some **guidelines** as to how you can best make the diagnosis of pulmonary tuberculosis. These include:

1.2.4 Symptoms (Figure 4 p 18)

Respiratory		*General*	
• • •	Cough	• •	Loss of weight
• • •	Sputum	• •	Fever and sweating
• •	Blood-spitting	•	Tiredness
•	Chest wall pain	•	Loss of appetite
•	Breathlessness		
•	Localised wheeze		
•	Frequent colds		

(The number of dots show which symptoms are most important.)

We must say a little more here about the above list of symptoms. All the symptoms could be due to other illnesses. To make sure, **you must examine the sputum for TB.**

One of the most important things which should make you think of possible tuberculosis is that the symptoms have **come on gradually over weeks or months.** This applies particularly to the **general symptoms of illness**: loss of weight, loss of appetite, tiredness or fever.

Cough, of course, is a common symptom after acute respiratory infections. It is also common in smokers. It is common in some areas where the houses or huts have no chimneys and the houses are often full of smoke – especially in cold climates or cold weather when fires may be used for heating as well as cooking. Both tobacco and domestic smoke lead to **chronic bronchitis**. Cough may come on gradually in a patient with **lung cancer**, which is becoming commoner in countries with increasing cigarette smoking. **Bronchiectasis** is common in some countries: the patient may have had a chronic cough with purulent sputum since childhood. But if a **patient has had a cough for more than 3 weeks you must get his sputum examined for TB** to make sure the cough is not due to tuberculosis. There is nothing in the **sputum** which itself suggests tuberculosis: it may be mucoid, purulent or contain blood. In tuberculosis, **blood in the sputum** may vary from a few spots to a sudden coughing of a large amount of blood. Occasionally this blood loss is so great that the patient quickly dies, usually from asphyxia due to aspirated blood. **If you see blood in the sputum you must always examine the sputum for TB**.

Pain in the chest is not uncommon in tuberculosis. Sometimes it is just a dull ache. Sometimes it is worse on breathing in (due to pleurisy). Sometimes it is due to muscle strain from coughing. Sometimes the cough has been so severe that the patient has cracked a rib (**cough fracture**).

Breathlessness in tuberculosis is due to extensive disease in the lungs, or to pleural effusion complicating the lung tuberculosis (p 104). The breathless patient frequently appears ill and has lost weight. He will often have fever.

Occasionally the patient has a **localised wheeze**. This is due to local tuberculous bronchitis or to pressure of a lymph node on a bronchus.

Sometimes the patient seems to have developed an acute **pneumonia**. But the pneumonia may not get better with routine antibiotics. The cough and fever may persist. The patient remains ill. If you question him closely you may find that he has had cough and loss of weight for weeks or months before the pneumonia came on. If there is any doubt **examine his sputum for TB**.

Sometimes the patient says that for months he has had one cold after another. Question him carefully. The colds may be just that a chronic cough has got repeatedly worse: **examine the sputum for TB**.

Remember that, in an older smoker, cough and loss of weight which come on gradually, may be due to **lung cancer**. But you **must** check for tuberculosis by examining the sputum.

Women who develop tuberculosis may lose their periods (**amenorrhoea**). They usually have other symptoms as well.

1.2.5 Physical signs. Often these do not help much. But do examine the patient carefully. You may find useful signs:

1. **General condition**. Sometimes this may be good, in spite of advanced disease. But the patient may be **obviously ill**. He may be **very thin**,

with obvious loss of weight. He may be **pale** or have a **flush** due to fever.

2. **Fever.** This can be of any type. There may be only slight rise of temperature in the evening. The temperature may be high or irregular. Often there is no fever.
3. **Pulse** is usually raised in proportion to fever.
4. **Finger clubbing.** You may find this, especially in a patient with extensive disease. Remember that clubbing is common with lung cancer.
5. **Chest.** Often there are no abnormal signs. The commonest is **fine crepitations** (crackles) in the upper part of one or both lungs. These are heard particularly on taking a deep breath after coughing. Later there may be **dullness to percussion** or even **bronchial breathing** in the upper part of both lungs. Occasionally there is a **localised wheeze** due to local tuberculous bronchitis or pressure by a lymph node on a bronchus. In chronic tuberculosis, with much fibrosis (scarring) the scarring may pull the trachea or the heart over to one side. At any stage the physical signs of pleural effusion (p 104) may be present. **But often you will find nothing abnormal in the chest.**

1.3   Investigations

1.3.1 **The most reliable way of making the diagnosis is to find TB in a direct smear of the sputum.** Examination is by the Ziehl–Neelsen (ZN) staining method or, in well equipped centres, by using modern fluoroscopy with ultraviolet light. Figure 25 is a flow chart as a guide to making the diagnosis.

In **collecting sputum for examination** you should make sure about the following:

1. The **containers** should be rigid to avoid crushing when carried or sent. They should be wide-mouthed. They should have tight fitting screw tops to prevent drying out and leakage. The method of **sterilisation** after use depends on the material the container is made of. Some can be burnt. Glass containers should be boiled for 10 minutes and then thoroughly cleaned.
2. Examine three specimens if possible:
   a) a **first spot** specimen when the patient presents himself
   b) an **early morning specimen** consisting of all the sputum raised in the first 1–2 hours
   c) a **second spot specimen** when the patient returns with the early morning specimen.
3. **Instructions to the technician for collection of sputum:**
   a) If possible do the procedure in the open air. If not, use a room set aside for this purpose.

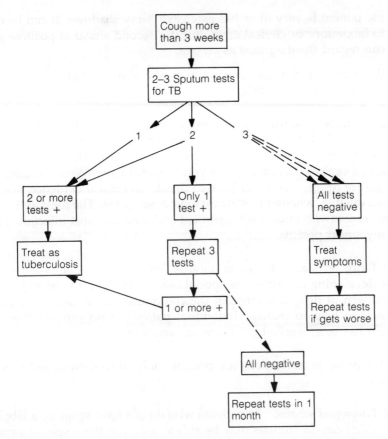

Figure 25 *Adult pulmonary tuberculosis: tuberculosis suspect.* Diagnostic flow chart

   b)   Explain why the test is important. Explain how to cough so as to produce sputum from deep in the chest.

   c)   Label the bottom part of the container (not the lid) with his name and number. Give him the bottom part. Keep the lid.

   d)   Stand behind the patient. Ask him to hold the container close to his lips, then cough and spit into it.

   e)   Check that the specimen has solid or purulent particles in it. If not, ask him to try again.

   f)   Close the container securely. Put it in a special box for the laboratory.

   g)   Wash your hands with soap and water.

   Keep a full and accurate **register of sputum examinations** (see reference 11, p 215). Make sure the specimens are properly labelled with the patient's name clearly marked.

4. Be careful about making a diagnosis on a single positive smear unless

the patient is very ill or has extensive X-ray shadows. It can be due to laboratory or clerical error. But if a second smear is positive you can regard the diagnosis as certain.

For the detailed techniques of sputum examination see the useful booklet given in reference 11, p 215.

1.3.2 Culture of sputum improves the number of positives, but it may take 4–8 weeks before you get the result. With milder disease and fewer TB the smears may be negative but culture positive. But culture needs skilled laboratory facilities which you may not have. While waiting for the culture result(s) you will have to decide on clinical evidence, and X-ray if available, whether to start treatment: see p 154. The illest and most severe cases (who most need treatment and who are most infectious) are usually smear positive.

1.3.3 Drug resistance tests can only be done in special laboratories. In most developing countries the special laboratory is best used to look at the pattern of drug resistance in the community. It should not usually be used to help to manage individual patients. Find out whether the pattern has been worked out for your own area.

The following investigations are possible only in well equipped special centres:

1.3.4 *Laryngeal swabs.* In patients who do not have sputum, a labora-tory which can do cultures may be able to give you these special swabs. The operator should wear a mask and gown when taking a swab: the patient's tongue is held using a piece of lint and the swab pushed down behind the tongue towards the larynx. The patient will cough and the swab will catch some mucus. Put the swab back into the sterile bottle and send to the laboratory for culture.

1.3.5 Gastric suction (often called 'gastric lavage' or 'washings'). This may be used when a patient has no sputum. It is only necessary if you have some difficult problem in diagnosis and if you have the facilities. It is sometimes used in children, who seldom produce sputum (Appendix F, p 206). In adults do gastric suction soon after the patient wakes and before he has had anything by the mouth. Pass a well lubricated fine nasogastric rubber tube through the nose to the back of the mouth. Then ask the patient to suck water through a 'straw' or fine tube. While he does this push the nasal tube gently in and it will pass easily into the stomach. Attach a syringe containing 20 ml of sterile normal saline through the nasogastric tube. Inject it slowly down the tube. Wait about a minute and then aspirate as much as possible back into the syringe.

Inject the contents into a sterile bottle and send to the laboratory. There it can be examined by smear and culture.

1.3.6 *Bronchoscopy*. When other methods have failed to make a diagnosis you may be able to collect bronchial material by a trap specimen through a bronchoscope. **Biopsy** of the lining of the bronchi may sometimes show typical changes of tuberculosis when examined by histology.

1.3.7 *Pleural fluid*. TB may occasionally be seen in centrifuged fluid but usually are only found on culture. The larger the amount of fluid cultured the more likely it is that you will get a positive.

1.3.8 Pleural biopsy can be useful when there is pleural effusion. But it needs a special biopsy needle (Abrams punch), facilities for histology and training in the technique. In many places none of these is available.

1.3.9 *Lung biopsy*. Only experienced operators should use this method. A diagnosis may be made by histology or by finding TB in the sections.

1.4 X-ray (radiological) examination

You cannot diagnose tuberculosis with certainty on an X-ray. Other diseases often look very similar.

1.4.1 A **normal chest X-ray** for practical purposes excludes tuberculosis. (Though very rarely tuberculosis causes tuberculous bronchitis which you cannot see on an X-ray.)

1.4.2 The X-ray shadows which strongly suggest tuberculosis are:

a) upper zone **patchy or nodular shadows** (on one or both sides), (e.g. Figure 23b, c and Figure 24a)
b) **cavitation** (particularly if more than one cavity) (Figure 23c, d)
c) **calcified shadows** may cause difficulties in diagnosis. Remember this may not be completely diagnostic. Pneumonia and lung tumours can occur in areas of previous healed and calcified tuberculosis. Some benign tumours contain calcification.

1.4.3 Other shadows which may be due to tuberculosis are:

a) **oval** or **round solitary shadow** (tuberculoma) (Figure 26a)
b) **hilar** and **mediastinal shadows** due to enlarged lymph nodes (persisting primary complex) (Figure 26b)
c) **diffuse small nodular shadows** (Figure 26c) (miliary tuberculosis: p 107).

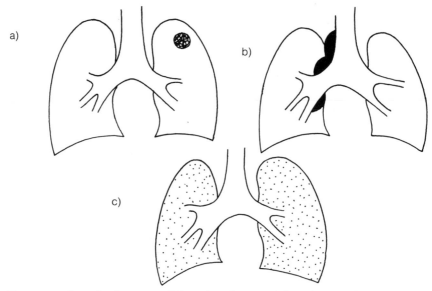

Figure 26 *Some further types of X-ray in pulmonary tuberculosis.* **a)** Rounded 'tub-erculoma' or coin lesion, upper zone of left lung. **b) Enlarged right hilar and paratracheal lymph nodes** of the primary complex (may be with or without obvious lung component). In an adult this appearance may look like a hilar carcinoma. Sometimes it is accompanied by high fever. This sort of appearance is very rare in adults of European origin, except in HIV victims, but may occur in adult Asians or Africans. **c)** The diffuse, evenly distributed, small nodular lesions of **miliary tuberculosis**. In the earliest stages these may be difficult to detect

The **correct reading of chest X-rays needs a lot of experience**.

If you suspect tuberculosis from the X-ray and the sputum is negative, give a non-tuberculosis antibiotic (e.g. ampicillin, oxytetracyline) for 7–10 days and repeat the X-ray. Shadows of an acute pneumonia will show improvement. But beware of shadows which look smaller after 10 days but are in fact due to collapse of part of the lung due to obstruction of a bronchus.

> IT IS A MAJOR ERROR TO DIAGNOSE TUBERCULOSIS ON X-RAY AND FAIL TO EXAMINE THE SPUTUM.

1.5   Tuberculin test

1.5.1   Technical details of tuberculin testing are given in Appendix E (p 200). Although, with proper attention to careful technique, tuberculin testing is very useful in measuring the prevalence of tuberculosis in a community, in many poorer countries it is much less valuable as a tool for diagnosis. This is because the test may be negative due to malnutrition or other diseases even though the patient has active tuberculosis. A strongly positive test is, of course, a point in favour of tuberculosis, but a negative test does not exclude tuberculosis. (Remember a strongly positive test is only a point in favour: many people without active tuberculosis have positive tests. In general the test is of little use for adults.)

1.5.2 There are two other problems in using the tuberculin test:

a) In many countries infection by other, often non-pathogenic, myco-bacteria can result in a positive tuberculin test, but usually a weak positive. A positive can also be due to previous BCG.
b) Problems of improper storage, improper dilution, absorption of tuberculin on to glass, contamination etc. may make the test unreliable in your area. We suggest you consult a local tuberculosis specialist who should be able to tell you whether the test will be valuable in your area.

But in any case remember that, **if other evidence suggests the diagnosis of tuberculosis, a negative test does NOT exclude tuberculosis**.

1.5.3 On the other hand a positive test, even a strongly positive test, only shows that the patient has previously been infected. It does not prove that he has active tuberculous disease. It is merely a point in favour. A positive test is particularly valuable in a young child at an age when fewer children in the community will normally have positive tests (p 46).

1.6 Blood examination

1.6.1 Marked **anaemia** is rarely caused by pulmonary tuberculosis but is sometimes seen in obscure ('cryptic') miliary tuberculosis (p 108). Anaemia is more likely to be due to other causes e.g. worms or malnutrition.

1.6.2 The **white blood count** is usually normal or low normal. (It is often raised in pneumonia.)

1.6.3 A raised **erythrocyte sedimentation rate** (ESR) may occur. But a normal result does not exclude active tuberculosis. It is therefore not a useful test and not worth doing.

1.6.4 Low serum potassium or sodium may occur in severe disease and can cause death. Many centres will not have facilities for these tests. If found, correct by intravenous drip.

Finally ALL PATIENTS PRESENTING WITH COUGH AND SPUTUM FOR MORE THAN 3 WEEKS MUST HAVE THEIR SPUTUM EXAMINED FOR TB.

1.7   Newer 'molecular' diagnostic methods

Much work is being done on methods to detect molecular components of TB in sputum. But so far these are not sufficiently straightforward or reliable for general use. The same applies to blood serum antibody tests. Similar methods are being developed for rapid drug resistance testing.

1.8   Distinguishing tuberculosis from other conditions

The main conditions which have to be distinguished are:

1.8.1 Pneumonia.   In acute pneumonia the symptoms usually come on suddenly. In the X-ray the soft shadows may look like tuberculosis. This is especially so if they are in the upper part of the lung. If the sputum is negative, give a non-tuberculous antibiotic for 7 days and X-ray again. A raised white blood count is in favour of pneumonia. If you have no X-ray, a rapid fall of temperature when you give the antibiotic makes the diagnosis likely to be pneumonia.

Pneumonia due to *Pneumocystis carinii* is a common complication of AIDS. There is often a low-grade fever for several weeks and cough without sputum. For details see chapter on HIV/TB p 142.

1.8.2 Lung cancer.   In the X-ray a tumour may sometimes break down into a cavity. Or infection beyond a bronchus blocked by a tumour may cause a lung abscess with a cavity. If the sputum is negative diagnosis may have to be made by bronchoscopy. A solid rounded tumour may be difficult to distinguish on the X-ray from a rounded tuberculous lesion. A patient with lung cancer is almost always a smoker. Feel also for an enlarged lymph node behind the inner end of the clavicle, a common place for secondary tumour.

1.8.3 Lung abscess.   There is usually a lot of purulent sputum. The patient is usually feverish and ill. If the purulent sputum is repeatedly negative for TB lung abscess is more likely. The white blood count is usually high.

1.8.4 Bronchiectasis.   There is usually a lot of purulent sputum. It has often been produced since childhood. Persistent moist coarse 'crackles' may be repeatedly heard over the same area of the lung. Sputum is negative for TB.

1.8.5 Asthma. Wheeze is not common in tuberculosis. But it may occasionally occur:

a) from enlarged lymph nodes, which may obstruct a bronchus or even the trachea,
b) from tuberculous bronchitis.

Either of these may cause a localised wheeze. Remember also that a few patients with severe asthma may be on **long-term corticosteroid drugs** (such as prednisolone). This can weaken the patient's defences against TB. He can then develop tuberculosis as well as asthma. **If an asthma patient develops a cough while under treatment, or if he begins to run a fever or loses weight, test his sputum for TB.**

SOME STORIES ABOUT DIAGNOSIS

A happy story

Mrs Kamal, a **20-year-old woman**, had recently married and had gone to live with her husband in his parents' house. A few months later she began to feel **tired**, lost her **appetite** and began to have a little **cough**. At first the family thought it was the strain of recent marriage. Then she lost her periods and they thought she might be pregnant. In the end her mother-in-law brought her up to the outpatient department of the **district hospital**. Her symptoms had now lasted 2 months. The doctor thought tuberculosis was a possibility. He asked if anyone else in the family had a cough. The mother-in-law said that her husband (the patient's father-in-law) had a chronic cough for a year or more and had lost some weight.

On **examination** the doctor found Mrs Kamal rather **thin**. She had a slight **fever**. He found **nothing else abnormal**. He asked her to cough up some **sputum** into a container. He gave her another container. He asked her to cough into it **first thing the next morning**, producing as much sputum as she could. He sent her to the X-ray department for a **chest X-ray**.

The doctor asked Mrs Kamal and her mother-in-law to come back the next morning with the sputum specimen. He would then tell them about the X-ray result. He asked the **mother-in-law to bring up her husband** at the same time so that he could find out the cause of the husband's cough.

The 'spot specimen' of sputum which Mrs Kamal had given in the clinic was negative. But the early morning sputum she produced next day was **positive for TB**. So as to make sure, the doctor asked for another early morning sputum which also turned out positive. The **X-ray** showed soft shadows in the right upper zone of the lung with a small cavity.

The **father-in-law's sputum** also proved **strongly positive** on two occasions. His chest X-ray was abnormal. Mrs Kamal's husband and her mother-in-law were well. They had no cough and no sputum to test. Their chest X-rays were clear.

The **doctor explained everything in a careful and friendly way** to the whole family. He told them all about the **treatment** and gave them each a leaflet to take home. Both patients took their treatment regularly and came back regularly for medicine. Both of them **soon lost their symptoms** and **felt very well**.

A year and a half later Mrs Kamal presented **her husband with a son**. The whole family came back to see the doctor and to thank him. The doctor arranged for the new son to have BCG as a precaution.

A more complicated story. The diagnosis nearly missed.

Mr Ram Musa, a **40-year-old man**, had been a farm worker. One year ago he had moved with his family to the city in search of a better life. Since then he had worked in a factory. He was only paid a small wage. This was not enough to give his family decent housing. He and his wife and three children lived in a hut he had built on waste ground.

Mr Musa was a heavy smoker. For some years he had had a '**smoker's cough**', worse in the morning. For the last 3 months his **cough had got worse**. He began to feel more **tired** than usual. His **appetite** became poorer. He thought he was getting **thinner**.

He first went to a **local healer**. The healer gave him medicine and charged him a fee. But Mr Musa got worse, not better. So he went to a **private doctor**, who gave him an antibiotic and charged him a fee. He went back to the doctor several times. The doctor gave him other medicines and charged him more fees. The patient continued to get worse.

Finally, feeling now very ill and having run out of money he went to a **government health centre** where there was a well-trained Health Assistant (HA). Because Mr Musa had a **chronic cough**, **loss of appetite** and **loss of weight**, the Health Assistant thought he might have tuberculosis. When he examined him he found that he was **thin** and had a **slight fever**. There were **no definite physical signs** in the chest. There was no X-ray machine at the health centre.

The HA asked Mr Musa to give a specimen of **sputum** right away. He gave him another sputum container and asked him to cough into it first thing the next morning and come back to the clinic. Both **specimens of sputum were positive for TB**.

The HA decided that he would start Mr Musa on **anti-tuberculosis chemotherapy** right away. In a **kind and friendly way** he told him the diagnosis and the treatment. He told him how long it would last and why. He gave him a **leaflet** to remind him of what he had been told. Mr Musa himself could not read: but his eldest 10-year-old son could and would be able to read the leaflet to him at home.

The HA asked Mr Musa to **come back next day with his wife and children**. When they came back he greeted them in a friendly way. He told the wife what he had already told the patient. He asked her to make sure that the patient took his treatment regularly. He asked her to make sure the patient came back to the clinic on the right date for further supplies. He told them both that if Mr Musa did not take his treatment regularly the tuberculosis might come back and kill him. He also told him that smoking **was bad for his health**. He said that if he stopped smoking it would help him to feel better quickly. It would also give him more money to support his family. If he took his treatment regularly he could continue to work, as otherwise the children would starve.

The HA examined **Mr Musa's wife and children**. They felt well. He found nothing obviously wrong. The children had been born in a remote country area and they had **not had BCG**: there was no scar on any of their arms. The HA gave the children and the wife **tuberculin tests**. He asked them to come back three days later when he read the tests (p 205). The test of the 10-year-old boy and the 7-year-old girl were **negative**. So the HA arranged for them to have BCG. The test of the 3-year old daughter was **strongly positive**. Because at that age there is a big risk of the child developing miliary tuberculosis (p 52) or tuberculous meningitis (p 58) after a tuberculous primary infection, the HA prescribed daily **isoniazid** for 6 months for this child (p 197).

The **wife** had a **weakly positive tuberculin test**. He asked her to come back at once if she developed a cough or felt ill in any way.

In any case she came back regularly with the 3-year-old child to get new supplies of isoniazid. He made sure that on each occasion both the child and the mother seemed well.

Mr Musa soon lost his cough, felt very much better and began to put on **weight**. He also stopped smoking. Two **sputa** were **negative** when tested after 2 months' treatment. He had no sputum to test after that. He was now feeling so much better that he was doing his work at the factory much better. So he was **given a better job** and got more money. He was also saving money by not smoking. So he was able to move his family into a **better home**. The **child remained well** after a year and was discharged from the clinic.

Comment: This is a common story. Mr Musa may have been **infected with TB when he came into the town**. There he lived in **bad conditions** and probably met **many people with infectious tuberculosis**. Or the bad conditions he was living in may have caused an **old primary infection** to break down.

In many countries patients will first go to local healers. In some places doctors have tried to encourage local healers to send patients to health clinics or health centres if they seem really ill or don't recover quickly. The **private doctor** should have had the patient's sputum examined for TB. Many private doctors fail to do this: it is very bad medicine.

The **Health Assistant** did his job very well. He immediately thought of tuberculosis. He immediately had the sputum examined. He gave the right treatment. He took time and trouble to explain everything in a friendly way both to the patient and his wife. He immediately looked for possible tuberculosis in the wife and children. He gave preventive treatment to the youngest child who had probably been recently infected by her father. He not only cured Mr Musa and his daughter from tuberculosis. He also helped him to stop smoking. So **everyone in the family ended up both well and also less poor.**

A wrong diagnosis

Mr Kozo Bang, a **20-year-old young man**, had a **smoker's cough**. One winter he had a **bad cold**. The **cough** got **worse** and he produced more **yellow sputum**. After 10 days he went to see a private doctor who sent him for an **X-ray**. He had to pay a fee for the doctor and he had to pay for the X-ray. The X-ray showed some soft shadows in the upper part of the left lung. The doctor **diagnosed tuberculosis**. He started Mr Bang on treatment with rifampicin and isoniazid. He **did not examine the sputum for TB**. Mr Bang soon felt rather better. But he only had enough money now to pay for 2 weeks' treatment. He did not have enough money to go back to the doctor. So he went to the outpatient department of the **District Hospital**. There the doctor **repeated the X-ray** and asked him to produce **two specimens of sputum** which he had examined for TB. The **X-ray was normal**. The two **sputa were negative**.

The doctor told Mr Bang that he did not have tuberculosis. He told him he had had a **mild pneumonia** which had now cleared up. But he strongly advised him to **stop smoking**. If he did not, he might easily get pneumonia again and could get other diseases also. Mr Bang stopped smoking, his cough disappeared completely and he continued to feel well.

Comment: You **cannot** diagnose tuberculosis with certainty on an X-ray. A pneumonia can look the same. **Many patients are given a lot of anxiety and take unnecessary anti-tuberculosis treatment for many months just because a doctor has made a diagnosis of tuberculosis on an X-ray and has failed to examine the sputum.** You **must examine the sputum for TB.** If it is negative in three specimens, repeat the X-ray in 4 weeks. If the shadows were due to pneumonia, they will improve or disappear in 2–3 weeks.

A case of 'pneumonia'

Mr Chowdhuri, a **man aged 50**, was admitted to a district hospital as a case of pneumonia. He had had a **bad cough** and felt **feverish** for 7–10 days. For 3 days he had had a **pain in the right side of his chest**, worse when he breathed in. The doctor found him **flushed**, **ill** and **obviously breathless**. He had a **high temperature** and a **fast pulse**. The doctor heard **crepitations** (crackles) scattered on both sides of the chest. He was unable to take a deep breath because of the pain in his right chest: the doctor could not hear a pleural rub. **X-ray of the chest** showed scattered soft shadows on both sides.

The doctor decided Mr Chowdhuri had bronchopneumonia and prescribed amoxycillin. After 5 days he was, if anything, worse. The doctor then questioned him carefully about his illness. Mr Chowdhuri said that for several months he had been feeling tired and had lost some weight. He had had a little cough. Ten days before he came into hospital these symptoms had begun to get much worse and he felt very feverish.

With this more detailed story, the doctor thought the illnesses could be tuberculosis. He sent two sputum specimens for examination for TB. They both came back positive.

When the doctor got the results of the sputum tests, he immediately put the patient on anti-tuberculosis chemotherapy. Within a few days there was great improvement. In 10 days the fever had subsided. Soon after that Mr Chowdhuri went home to continue his treatment. In due course he recovered completely.

Comment: Occasionally a patient with tuberculosis may seem to have an acute pneumonia, but fails to improve with pneumonia treatment. If you question him closely you will often find that he has had some symptoms for weeks or months before these became more acute and brought him to hospital.

1.9 Complications

1.9.1 Pleurisy and empyema are discussed on p 104.

1.9.2 Spontaneous pneumothorax occurs when air escapes into the pleural space following rupture of a tuberculous cavity. This causes sudden acute chest pain on that side together with breathlessness. It may go on to **tuberculous empyema** (p 104).

1.9.3 Tuberculous laryngitis is described on p 115.

1.9.4 Cor pulmonale (congestive cardiac failure due to back pressure from damaged lung) may occur if there is very extensive destruction of the lungs. This may happen even if the tuberculous disease is no longer active, but has left a lot of scarring. Early treatment of tuberculosis obviously makes this less likely.

1.9.5 Aspergillomata. Well treated and 'healed' tuberculous cavities sometimes remain open and can be infected by the fungus *Aspergillus fumigatus*. On the X-ray you may see a ball of fungus within the cavity. This sometimes causes severe, and even fatal, haemoptysis (coughing up

blood). If bleeding keeps on recurring, and you have got surgical facilities, you may have to consider resecting the cavity. But often the patient's lung function has been too much damaged by the old tuberculosis so that he is not fit for operation.

2: TUBERCULOUS PLEURAL EFFUSION AND EMPYEMA

2.1   How the pleura is affected

The pleura, which is part of the respiratory system, may be affected in three different ways:

1.   Effusion which develops within a few months of primary infection (p 31) in children and young adults.
2.   Effusion developing as a result of lung disease in older adults. Rarely this may go on to a purulent effusion (**empyema**).
3.   Rupture of a tuberculous cavity and escape of air into the pleural space. This allows air to escape into the space between the lung and the chest wall. The TB from the ruptured cavity produce a purulent effusion (**empyema**). The air and the pus together are called a **pyopneumothorax**.

2.2   How it shows clinically

1.   Pain when the patient breathes in (pleuritic pain) which later becomes a dull ache in the lower chest.
2.   Fever which may be mild and not last long.
3.   Slight irritating cough.
4.   Breathlessness on exertion.
5.   Dullness to percussion over the lower part of the chest.
6.   No sounds of air entry when you listen over that area of the chest.
7.   In large effusions the mediastinum is pushed away from the affected side (Figure 27).
8.   Tuberculin test is sometimes negative especially if malnourished, recent measles, or HIV infected. If negative at first, it may prove positive if you repeat it a month later.
9.   There may be an abscess over the lower chest if the empyema spreads through the chest wall between the ribs. (Remember that a 'cold' fluctuant swelling – not hot or tender – can be due to a 'cold abscess'

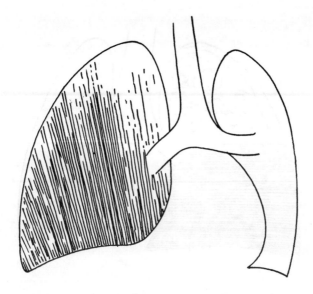

Figure 27 *Large right pleural effusion.* Note that the trachea, heart and medias-tinum are pushed over to the left

from a tuberculous intercostal lymph node or an abscess tracking round the chest wall from a tuberculous spine (p 63).)

2.3 How to investigate it

2.3.1 X-ray of the chest (Figure 27). Large effusions are most dense at the base, thinner at the top. You cannot see the diaphragm. But the shadow thins out at the top. If you are not sure whether fluid is present, take another X-ray with the patient supine (lying down flat on his back). The fluid shadow will move.

If a cavity has burst, air as well as liquid will be present. The top of the fluid will be flat, with the air above it (Figure 28). This gives a splashing sound if you shake the chest.

2.3.2 Remove some fluid with a syringe and needle (or by intercostal tube if the pus is too thick). Send the fluid or pus for examination for TB.

2.3.3 If you have the facilities and the training, at the same time remove a piece of pleura tissue (biopsy) (p 95). Send this for examination under the microscope (histology).

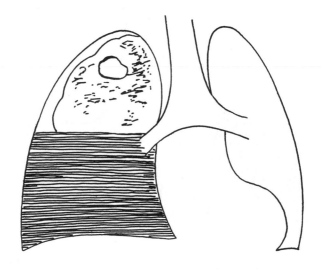

Figure 28 *A cavity has burst into the pleura.* Air as well as fluid is present. So the top of the fluid will be flat. The fluid often turns to pus (**pyopneumothorax**)

2.4   Other conditions which have to be distinguished

1. Tumour
2. Other infections (e.g. pneumonia; pleural fluid resulting from amoebic abscess of the liver, if on right side)
3. Heart disease
4. Pulmonary embolism and infarction

2.5   Management

1. Chemotherapy as detailed on p 165 and 174.
2. If possible prednisolone as detailed on p 188.
3. Aspiration (drawing off) of fluid: this will probably only be required once. There is usually rapid response to treatment.
4. (Sometimes it may be necessary to remove a localised empyema by operation.)

2.6   End result

This is usually satisfactory. But, if neglected, the pleura may become very thick and fibrotic. This can cause shrinkage of the chest wall and later breathlessness.

3: MILIARY TUBERCULOSIS IN ADULTS

3.1 How it arises

Miliary tuberculosis is due to spread through the blood stream of large numbers of TB which the patient's defences are too weak to kill off. (It is called 'miliary' because the small lesions in the organs seemed to 19th century pathologists to look like millet seeds.) TB may enter the blood by:

1. Spread to the blood stream from a **recent primary infection**. This may occur by way of the lymph nodes and lymphatics or by a tuberculous lesion eroding a blood vessel.
2. **Reactivation of an old tuberculous lesion** (primary or post-primary) with erosion of a blood vessel. Reactivation may occur if the patient's defences are lowered, for instance by HIV infection, another disease, malnutrition or old age.
3. Spread into the blood stream after a **surgical operation** on an organ containing a tuberculous lesion. (Always give chemotherapy before and after the operation.)

3.2 Why diagnosing it is particularly important

If not properly treated almost all patients will die. If properly treated almost all patients should recover. If you can get an X-ray of the chest, the diagnosis may be quite easy, but in some cases it can be very difficult. The X-ray may fail to show the lesions. In some places no X-ray may be available. Moreover, particularly in the elderly, the disease may be much less acute ('cryptic miliary tuberculosis': *see below*) and it is easy to forget the possibility.

3.3 How it shows clinically in adults

Clinically the patients may be divided into three different types (Table 6).

3.3.1 **'Classical'** miliary tuberculosis. There is a history of gradual onset of **fever**, malaise and loss of weight, usually over weeks. It may follow some other illness, e.g. measles. There is nothing typical about the kind of fever, which varies widely. There may be evidence of a **tuberculous lesion** somewhere in the body, but often this is not obvious. Sometimes there is enlargement of the **liver** or **spleen** (though less often than in children) – but of course there are many other reasons for this.

If you have an ophthalmoscope look for **choroidal tubercles** (p 71). These are seen less often in adults than in children but if present make the diagnosis certain. Check for neck stiffness and other signs of

Table 6   *Summary of types of miliary tuberculosis in adults*

	Acute 'Classical'	Cryptic	'Non-reactive'
Frequency	Common	Rare	Now less rare: HIV
Age	Any age	Usually elderly	Any age
Fever, malaise, loss of weight	Prominent	Mild	Usually desperately ill
Choroidal tubercles	15–30%	Absent	? Absent
Meningitis	10%	May be terminal	Absent
Enlargement of liver/spleen	May be present	Rare	May be present
Chest X-ray	Usually miliary shadows	No shadows at first	May or may not be shadows
Tuberculin test	Positive or negative	Often negative	Usually negative
Blood abnormality	May be anaemia etc.	Often anaemia	May be anaemia (often aplastic), pancytopenia, agranulocytosis, leukaemoid reaction
Low serum sodium/ potassium	Especially elderly and women	Normal	?
Diagnostic biopsy	Seldom needed	Often helps	Diagnostic: especially bone marrow

meningeal irritation (p 58): **tuberculous meningitis** often complicates miliary tuberculosis.

X-ray of chest may show diffuse, evenly distributed, small shadows. They vary in different cases from vague shadows 1–2 mm in diameter to large dense shadows 5–10 mm in diameter. In the early stages of the illness none may be visible. If you do suspect miliary, take a dark (penetrating) X-ray and shine a bright light behind the outer rib spaces: this may show the first small lesions. The **white blood count** is usually normal or low. The **tuberculin test** may be negative. Without treatment **death** usually follows in weeks, but sometimes only after 1–3 months.

3.3.2 'Cryptic' (obscure) miliary tuberculosis. This usually occurs in the elderly. The **fever** is often mild or irregular. It may continue over months. There is often **anaemia**. There are usually no other helpful physical signs. The diagnosis is easy if the **chest X-ray** shows miliary lesions. But often at first it does not. Lesions may only appear after weeks or months. The **tuberculin test** is usually negative. Without treatment the patient slowly gets worse over months and eventually dies, with or without terminal meningitis.

3.3.3 Non-reactive miliary tuberculosis. Until the HIV epidemic arose this was very rare. It is now not uncommon in HIV infected patients. It is an acute malignant form of tuberculous septicaemia (spread of large numbers of TB through the blood stream). **Histologically** (under the microscope) the lesions are necrotic, not typical of tuberculosis, but with very large numbers of TB. The patient is extremely ill. The **chest X-ray** may or may not show lesions. The **tuberculin test** is negative. There are often **blood abnormalities**. These may include anaemia (often aplastic), pancytopenia (especially leucopenia or agranulocytosis) or appearances similar to leukaemia. The diagnosis is often missed. If so, the patient dies rapidly. The correct diagnosis may only be made at post mortem.

3.4 How to diagnose miliary tuberculosis

3.4.1 In tropical countries fever is common. Finding the cause is probably one of your commonest jobs. Make sure you always remember the possibility of miliary tuberculosis. For your patient it may make the difference between life and death.

3.4.2 If the history suggests that fever has been present for more than 7–10 days (which will exclude most of the acute infections), you must think of the possiblity of miliary. You must have a routine for investigating PUOs (Pyrexia or fevers of Unknown Origin). Your routine will partly depend on the common causes in your area and partly on your facilities for investigation (e.g. white blood counts, blood cultures and X-ray).

3.4.3 X-ray. If you can get a chest X-ray, this may be virtually diagnostic (3.3.1 above). Viral or bacterial pneumonia occasionally looks like miliary, but the shadows are likely to improve within a week or so under treatment for pneumonia. But, as we have already pointed out, a normal X-ray does not exclude miliary.

3.4.4 Sputum smear is usually negative. Culture if possible (though the result will come back too late to help you). Urine culture may also be positive in due course.

3.4.5 *Other specific investigations.* These are only needed in a difficult case.

If you have the facilities, **liver** or **bone marrow biopsy** may show

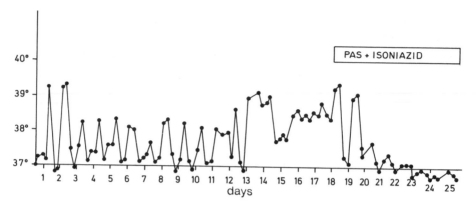

Figure 29 *Cryptic miliary tuberculosis* diagnosed because he improved with specific anti-tuberculosis treatment. Man aged 70 with continued fever, anaemia, a negative tuberculin test and no direct evidence of miliary tuberculosis: no abnormal clinical signs and an apparently normal chest X-ray. Usual investigations for fever of unknown origin negative. Using treatment with PAS and isoniazid (which would not affect other infections) his temperature fell and his blood count returned to normal

miliary tubercles on histology. If possible make sure part of the specimen is put in a **sterile container** (no preservative: this would kill TB) and sent for culture for TB. The result of culture will arrive too late to influence a decision about treatment, but may later confirm your diagnosis.

3.4.6 If the diagnosis is not clear clinically, if the chest X-ray is negative and you have no other means of diagnosis try the effect of **anti-tuberculosis treatment**. For this trial it is important to use **only drugs specific for tuberculosis** i.e. isoniazid (p 179) combined with thioacetazone (p 184) or ethambutol (p 183). For **diagnostic** purposes do **not** use streptomycin or rifampicin. These affect many other infections besides tuberculosis.

If the disease is tuberculosis, the fever will usually begin to come down within a week (Figure 29).

If you have decided the disease is tuberculosis, put the patient on full anti-tuberculosis treatment (p 153).

3.5   How to treat it

3.5.1 Acute and cryptic miliary tuberculosis respond well to standard chemotherapy. Fever and malaise usually begin to come down within days (occasionally longer) but it is usually a month or more before the X-ray starts to clear.

3.5.2 If the patient is **desperately ill** (with either acute or the rare non-reactive tuberculosis), and you have the facilities, it is justified to give **prednisolone** (p 188) with your chemotherapy. This will reduce the life-threatening toxicity and give the anti-tuberculosis drugs time to act. But it is dangerous to use prednisolone unless you are sure of the diagnosis (in case you are suppressing the patient's defences against some undiagnosed infection you are not treating). For obvious reasons you must not give prednisolone if you are using treatment for diagnosis (3.4.6).

TWO STORIES ABOUT MILIARY TUBERCULOSIS

A patient coming to a moderately well-equipped District Hospital
Mr Wong Fan, a **man aged 18**, came to the outpatient department. He looked **very ill**. He had a **high temperature**. He said that he had begun to feel **tired** about a month before. This had got steadily worse. He felt more and more ill. He felt **feverish** and **sweated a lot**. He lost his **appetite**. He was getting **thinner**. He had had a **slight cough** for several weeks. He had no other symptoms.

Because he looked so ill, the outpatient doctor immediately **admitted** him to a ward. There the doctor found a few **crepitations** (crackles) on each side of the chest. He could just feel the tip of the **spleen**. There was no neck stiffness, no rash, no enlarged lymph nodes. The doctor knew that malaria was frequent in the area, so many patients had an enlarged spleen. The story seemed a long one for typhoid. **Miliary tuberculosis** must be a possibility. He asked about cough or tuberculosis in the **family**. The patient said there was none.

To look for evidence of miliary tuberculosis the doctor dilated the pupils with eye drops. With his ophthalmoscope he carefully searched each retina for **choroidal tubercles** (p 71). He found two small, yellowish slightly raised areas near a blood vessel in the left retina. These were typical of choroidal tubercles. This made the diagnosis nearly certain. But he also got an **X-ray** of the chest. This showed widespread 4–5 mm rounded shadows throughout both lungs.

To be on the safe side the doctor sent 3 **blood smears** for **malaria** parasites. He also ordered **3 sputum examinations for TB** (culture for TB was not available). The blood smears were negative for malaria. There was very little mucoid sputum: these smears were negative for TB.

Because he had found the choroidal tubercles, the doctor did not wait for the results of these investigations. **He started the patient right away on anti-tuberculosis chemotherapy**.

Mr Wong Fan's **temperature began to come down** within 3 days. He felt much better and began to eat well. After 10 days the temperature was normal and he was gaining weight.

He was then **sent home** to continue his treatment and come up for regular checks and new supplies of drugs.

Before he left the doctor **carefully explained to him about the disease**. He also gave him a **leaflet** which explained the treatment. He explained to the family at the same time. He told them both that the **patient's life depended** on his taking every dose of the treatment for the full time. Otherwise the disease might come back and kill him. While Mr Wong Fan was in hospital the doctor **checked his parents and 3 siblings for tuberculosis**: none was found.

Comment: This was a **straightforward case**. With an ophthalmoscope and an X-ray it was easy to investigate **because the doctor thought about tuberculosis**. So he looked for **choroidal tubercles**. So he got an **X-ray of the chest**. But remember that many patients with miliary tuberculosis will **not** have choroidal tubercles. Remember also that **in the early stages miliary shadows may not show on the chest X-ray**. Remember that in miliary tuberculosis the **sputum is often negative** on direct smear. It is often positive on culture. But culture may not be available; in any case you would have to decide about treatment before you got the result.

A patient attending a rural health post with few facilities

Mrs Mawi, a **married woman aged 23**, had been **feverish** and **ill** for the last 10 days. She went to a local healer. He gave her medicine but she went on getting worse. She was now so ill that she had to be carried to the health post. She had **headache** with the fever but no other symptoms; no cough, no urinary symptoms, no diarrhoea.

The **Health Assistant** (HA) found that she was thin and ill. She had a **high temperature**. He found nothing abnormal in the chest. He could not feel the spleen or liver. There was no rash. There was no neck stiffness. He had no ophthalmoscope. He had not been trained to use one.

The HA examined a **blood slide for malaria**: it was negative. The patient had no sputum to examine. He thought she might have **enteric** (typhoid or paratyphoid) or perhaps **some other infection** or **miliary tuberculosis**. He asked about tuberculosis or whether any of the family had a chronic cough. They said that everyone else was well. He decided to give **chloramphenicol** first. This would deal with enteric and some other bacterial infections. If she was no better in 3 days he would add anti-tuberculosis chemotherapy. He could not refer her to hospital. The nearest was a day's walk. There was no road and no transport. She was obviously not fit to make the journey. Mrs Mawi lived close to the health post. Because she was so ill **3 days later** the HA went to see her at home. She said she was no better; indeed she was **worse**.

She was now so ill that he decided he could wait no longer. He **added anti-tuberculosis chemotherapy**. To be on the safe side he continued chloramphenicol also for a further 10 days. He did this in case she had enteric but was slow in improving with treatment. To be on the safe side he also took another **blood smear for malaria**. This was negative.

Next day she was a little better. **Three days later** she was definitely **feeling better** and her **temperature was lower**.

She gradually recovered completely. The HA carefully explained the importance of taking all the treatment for the full period, even after she was feeling entirely well. He also explained this to the family.

Although the **family** had said that everyone else was well, the HA when he visited the home noticed that the patient's **mother-in-law had a cough**. She said that she had had this for a year or more, but did not feel ill. The HA arranged for **3 sputum tests** for TB. Two of these were **positive**. So he also successfully treated her.

Mrs Mawi's two children, aged 3 and 5, had had **BCG** when they were infants. There were BCG scars on their arms. No tuberculin was available. They were well, but clearly had been at major risk of infection. So he arranged for them both to have 6 months of preventive INH. If they or the husband or the father-in-law became unwell they should come up at once. But all remained well.

Comment: Where there are few facilities the doctor or HA has to do his best with what he has got. He has to look for **clues in the patient's story**. In particular ask about **family illness which could be tuberculosis**. But if you can get no help from the story or physical signs you may have to **use treatment as a test of diagnosis**. Of course this can never be a certain test. The patient might be getting better from something else on his own. But it is the best you can do.

In this patient it might have been better to **continue the chloramphenicol for a week before deciding that it had failed**. But the patient was getting rapidly worse. The HA rightly decided that it was too big a risk to wait. So he **added anti-tuberculosis treatment**. The patient rapidly improved. This made tuberculosis very probable. The improvement **might** have been a delayed effect of the chloramphenical. But miliary tuberculosis is fatal without proper treatment. So it was much safer to treat it as miliary.

Note that the family had denied other illness. But the HA was sufficiently alert to spot the **mother-in-law's cough**. When he found her sputum positive this **strongly confirmed the diagnosis** in the original patient.

4
Non-pulmonary Tuberculosis in Adults

1: TUBERCULOSIS OF UPPER RESPIRATORY TRACT: EPIGLOTTIS, LARYNX, PHARYNX

Nearly all tuberculosis of the upper respiratory tract is a complication of pulmonary disease. (But blood-borne infection occasionally causes laryngeal tuberculosis with little to find elsewhere. Laryngeal tuberculosis has often been wrongly diagnosed as cancer of the larynx.) The epiglottis is often involved in laryngeal tuberculosis. The pharynx may also be affected.

1.1 How it shows clinically

1. The patient may have had **cough** and **sputum** for some time as laryngeal disease occurs most often in advanced pulmonary tuberculosis. There may also be **loss of weight**.
2. **Hoarseness** and changes in voice, becoming a moist whisper.
3. **Pain** in the **ear**.
4. **Pain** on **swallowing** which usually means the epiglottis is also involved. Pain may be severe.
5. In very advanced disease the **tongue** may also show ulcers.
6. Examination shows **ulceration of the cords** or other areas in the upper respiratory tract.
7. Examine the **sputum** for TB.
8. **X-ray** the chest if possible.

1.2 Distinguishing it from other diseases

The main disease to distinguish from tuberculosis is cancer. Malignant disease of the larynx is rarely painful. The sputum is usually positive but the diagnosis may need to be made by biopsy in difficult cases. If you cannot do a biopsy and you think tuberculosis is possible, try the effect of chemotherapy.

1.3   Management

Tuberculosis of the larynx responds extremely well to chemotherapy. If there is severe pain which does not quickly clear with treatment, add prednisolone (p 188) for 2–3 weeks (if available).

2: TUBERCULOSIS OF MOUTH, TONSIL AND TONGUE

Tuberculosis of the mouth is rare. It usually occurs in the **gum**. It shows as a relatively painless swelling which is often ulcerated. As it is frequently a primary lesion there is often enlargement of the regional lymph nodes. Both this and **tonsillar lesions**, which are similar, are likely to be due to infected milk, or perhaps occasionally food, or infected droplets from the air. Tonsillar lesions may not be obvious clinically.

Lesions of the **tongue** are usually secondary to advanced pulmonary tuberculosis. They are often ulcerated and may be very **painful**. They rapidly improve with chemotherapy.

3: TUBERCULOUS MENINGITIS

Tuberculous meningitis remains a major problem and an important cause of death in some countries. Human *Mycobacterium tuberculosis* is now responsible for most cases of tuberculous meningitis but opportunistic mycobacteria may cause the disease in patients with AIDS (p 135).

3.1   How it arises

In the course of spread from the primary tuberculous focus, or as part of miliary tuberculosis spread, tiny tubercles are seeded into the brain and meninges. Occasionally they may also be seeded into the bones of the skull or the vertebrae. These tubercles may rupture into the subarachnoid space and there cause:

1. **inflammation of the meninges**
2. **formation of a grey jelly-like mass at the base of brain**, and
3. **inflammation and narrowing of the arteries** leading to the brain which may cause local brain damage.

These three processes cause the clinical picture.

3.2 How it shows in the patient

There is usually a history of **general ill-health for 2–8 weeks** – malaise, tiredness, irritability, changes in behaviour, loss of appetite, loss of weight and mild fever. Then, as a result of:

1. **Inflammation of the meninges,** there will be headaches, vomiting and neck stiffness.
2. The **grey exudate involving the base of the brain** may affect the cranial nerves giving some of the expected signs: deterioration of vision, paralysis of an eyelid, squint, unequal pupils, deafness. Papilloedema is present in 40 per cent of patients.
3. **Involvement of the arteries** to the brain can lead to fits, loss of speech or loss of power in a limb or limbs. But any area of the brain may be damaged.
4. Some degree of **hydrocephalus** is common. This is due to blocking by exudate of some of the cerebrospinal fluid connections within the brain. Hydrocephalus is the main reason for decrease of consciousness. The resulting damage may be permanent and probably accounts for the bad prognosis in patients who are only seen when they are already unconscious.
5. **Spinal block** by exudate may cause upper motor neurone weakness or paralysis of the legs.
6. As **tuberculous disease elsewhere in the body** is often present look for:
   - tuberculosis of the lymph nodes
   - X-ray evidence of lung disease especially miliary tuberculosis (p 107) (if X-ray available)
   - enlargement of liver and/or spleen
   - (choroidal) tubercles visible on examination of the retina (p 71).

The **tuberculin test** may be negative especially in the advanced stages of the disease.

3.3 Diagnosis

The main conditions to be distinguished are bacterial meningitis, viral meningitis, and HIV-related cryptococcal meningitis. In the first two of these the onset is much more acute. Cryptococcal meningitis may have a much slower onset. A family history of tuberculosis, or the finding of tuberculosis somewhere else in the body, makes tuberculosis much more likely. But the best evidence comes from examination of the cerebrospinal fluid (CSF) obtained by lumbar puncture. The points are as follows:

1. **Pressure:** usually raised.
2. **Appearance:** at first looks clear but may form a 'spider's web' clot on standing. May be yellowish if there is spinal block.

3. **Cells**: 200–800 per mm³: many neutrophils at first (but not all neutrophils as in bacterial meningitis, which has a much higher cell count). Mainly lymphocytes later. The count may be low in AIDS.
4. **Glucose**: low in 90 per cent of patients, but may be normal in the early stage of the disease or in AIDS. This is very helpful in differentiating from viral meningitis in which the glucose is normal.
5. **Bacteriology**: smear positive only in 10 per cent unless large volume (10–12 ml) centrifuged long and hard. If the microscopist spends 30 minutes or more on a thick smear slide, then up to 90 per cent positives can be reached. Culture should be carried out if possible. It is usually positive, but can only give late confirmation of your diagnosis. Bacteriological diagnosis may obviously be made by obtaining mycobacteria from other specimens, e.g. sputum, pus. In HIV areas do Indian ink stain for cryptococci.

Prognosis: Death is certain if the disease is untreated: the earlier it is diagnosed and treated, the more likely is the patient to recover without serious permanent damage. The clearer the state of consciousness when treatment is started, the better the prognosis. If the patient is comatose the prognosis for complete recovery is poor. Unfortunately 10–30 per cent of survivors are left with some damage.

Because of the fatal outlook if diagnosis is missed TREAT IF THE DIAGNOSIS IS AT ALL LIKELY: for details of treatment see p 176.

4: TUBERCULOSIS OF THE PERICARDIUM

This is rare in many parts of the world and relatively common in others, especially where HIV infection is widespread.

4.1 How it arises

The bacilli may reach the pericardium through the blood (when there may be disease also in other organs). But it is more commonly due to rupture of a mediastinal lymph node into the pericardial space (p 34). It is rare for tuberculosis of the lungs to be present at the same time.

4.2 How it shows in the patient (clinical features)

Dry pericarditis shows by:

1. acute pain which the patient feels behind the sternum – it may be made better by sitting forward;

2. friction rub heard with the stethoscope over the heart and in time with the heart beat;
3. if you can get an electrocardiogram (ECG) you are likely to see widespread T-wave changes.

When **pericardial effusion** develops, the clinical signs are:

1. breathlessness on exertion (or even at rest);
2. a rapid pulse, which is paradoxical: big fall in blood pressure and pulse pressure on inspiration; this is not always present (this is because normally the negative pressure in the thorax on inspiration draws blood from the great veins into the heart – this is prevented if there is much fluid in the pericardium);
3. low blood pressure (sometimes severe);
4. raised jugular venous pressure;
5. enlarged liver;
6. fluid in the abdomen;
7. fever (of variable degree);
8. the friction rub may disappear as fluid develops but it sometimes continues.

X-ray examination usually shows a large pericardial effusion (see Figure 15, p 39).

The **tuberculin test** is usually positive.

Constrictive pericarditis: The inflammation of the pericardium may make it thicker and even calcified. **Calcification** may show on the X-ray as a narrow irregular white rim along the edge of the heart shadow (Figure 30). The thickened pericardium may form a sort of armour or casing over the heart. This may prevent it dilating in diastole (the expansion of the heart which sucks in the blood). The result is that the heart cannot take in enough blood from the veins.

The constriction may occur within months or weeks of the effusion. Sometimes it only shows itself years later, perhaps with no history suggesting a previous pericardial effusion.

The patient may come with:

1. **Breathlessness**. As the lungs are not congested the patient can lie down without increased breathlessness. There is no pulmonary oedema so **no** diffuse pulmonary crepitations.
2. There is **oedema** of legs etc., owing to back pressure in the systemic veins.
3. The **liver** may be very large. There may be ascites. The spleen may be enlarged.
4. The **heart is small and quiet**. This is quite different from most causes of congestive cardiac failure which have a large heart.
5. The **jugular venous pressure rises** with inspiration (normally, of course, it falls).

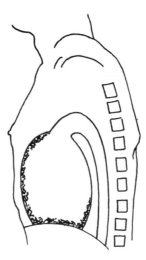

Figure 30 *Constrictive pericarditis.* Lateral X-ray film showing **thickening and calcification of the pericardium**. This 'armour' prevents full dilatation of the heart

6.   There is **paradoxical pulse** (see above).
7.   Look for signs of tuberculosis elsewhere in the body.

Most cases of constrictive pericarditis are due to tuberculosis. It is particularly suggested by the **small heart**, in spite of marked evidence of **oedema** in the limbs **without** congestion in the lungs. If possible take penetrating (black) X-rays which may show up the calcification which confirms the diagnosis.

4.3   Diagnosis

Diagnosis of tuberculous pericarditis is made by:

1.   evidence of **tuberculosis elsewhere** in the body,
2.   culture of pericardial fluid, if this is possible (60 per cent positive),
3.   biopsy of pericardium, if this is possible (70 per cent positive).

It has to be distinguished from disease of the heart muscle, other causes of heart failure and malignant disease.

4.4   Treatment

The disease responds well to standard chemotherapy (p 165). If possible **prednisolone** 30 mg twice daily for 4 weeks; reduced to 15 mg for next

4 weeks; then reduce dose slowly. This reduces the need for frequent aspirations of fluid and reduces the death rate.

Open drainage is rarely required.

Surgical removal of the pericardium is sometimes needed if constriction occurs. But try the effect of chemotherapy first. It may be effective. If surgery is not possible, chemotherapy is the best you can do.

A CASE OF TUBERCULOSIS PERICARDITIS IN A BOY AGED 9½ YEARS

Four months previously Tomas had developed **erythema nodosum** (p 131). At that time the doctor thought that this was connected with rheumatic fever. He had been put to bed and given salicylates for 6 weeks and kept away from school for 3 months.

Four days before he was admitted to hospital Tomas had again become **feverish** and **listless** and had complained of a **vague pain** in the upper part of his left arm and shoulder, later across the top of his chest. Next day the doctor heard a **pericardial friction rub**. He thought this was the result of rheumatic fever and sent Tomas to hospital. On **examination** Tomas was thin, wanting to lie still but not unduly ill or distressed. **Temperature** 39°C, **respiration rate** 24 and **pulse** 120. There was a marked **increase in cardiac dullness** particularly on the left side. There was a loud **pericardial friction rub** through which the heart sounds could be faintly heard. There was no heart murmur. The liver was not enlarged. The neck veins were not distended. In the chest there was some dullness and decreased air entry at the left base behind.

Diagnosis: Because of the erythema nodosum and the presence of a pericardial effusion in a boy who was not as ill as he would have been with rheumatic carditis the doctor thought of the possibility of tuberculosis. So he began **anti-tuberculosis chemotherapy** and then went on with the investigations. The **tuberculin test** was strongly positive. WBC 8000, Hb 110 per cent, both unlikely in acute rheumatism. Electrocardiogram was normal. **X-ray** showed a large heart shadow consistent with a pericardial effusion (see Figure 15, p 39) and some pleural reaction at the left base. Nothing abnormal was seen in the lung fields.

Within 4 days of starting treatment improvement had begun. His temperature subsided. Although the friction rub remained for 10 days the heart sounds became louder and were normal. **X-ray** on the 10th day confirmed that the effusion was smaller and it had disappeared in a third film taken after a month. But in the second and third X-rays there was evidence of enlargement of the **right hilar lymph nodes**. Three years later X-rays showed calcification in this area. He made a complete recovery.

Tomas's family were investigated. His parents were normal and his brother's tuberculin test was negative, but his **maternal grandfather** was found to have active pulmonary tuberculosis.

5: LYMPH NODE TUBERCULOSIS

5.1   General comments

Lymph node tuberculosis in adults is similar to lymph node tuberculosis in children, as described on p 56. But a few points are worth emphasising.

1. In older adults remember the possibility that enlarged nodes may be due to deposits of **carcinoma** coming from a primary carcinoma in the draining area. Hard nodes behind the inner end of the clavicle are often linked with a lung cancer. In some countries this will become more and more common as the tobacco smoking habit spreads.
2. In adults, as in children, there is usually no **fever** with tuberculous peripheral lymph nodes. But sometimes there is low fever. Occasionally we have seen very **high fever** in adults whose chest X-ray shows enlarged lymph nodes at the hilum and along the trachea. There may also be enlarged lymph nodes in the neck.

The **prognosis** is good as far as survival is concerned. But if there have been many discharging sinuses, these may result in much scarring.

The **tuberculin test** is usually positive, but may be negative if there is malnutrition etc. (p 46).

5.2   Treatment

Standard chemotherapy should be given as detailed on p 165. **Caution:** you never quite know what the lymph nodes will do when you treat them. In about a quarter of patients they may enlarge under treatment. New nodes may even appear. In about 20 per cent an abscess may develop and sometimes sinuses will form. All this is probably a hypersensitivity reaction to the tuberculin released from the killed bacilli. **Don't change treatment if this happens.** The nodes will subside if you continue the treatment as before.

In about 5 per cent of patients you may still be able to feel nodes at the end of treatment but usually they do not give further trouble. It is not necessary to give **prednisolone** (p 188) as a routine. But if there is a large fluctuant abscess, prednisolone may prevent sinuses and help the abscess to subside without having to use surgery. Do use prednisolone, if available, if there are massive mediastinal nodes. It helps them to subside more quickly. **Aspiration of abscesses** should be avoided if possible because sinuses may develop (if only rarely) in the needle track. It is better to make a small surgical incision and let out the pus.

In the old days a lot of **surgery** was done on tuberculous lymph nodes, with many operations for removal. With chemotherapy this is no longer necessary. The only reason to remove a node is if you have serious doubts about the diagnosis.

6: TUBERCULOSIS OF BONES AND JOINTS

Because the problems are so similar in adults to those in children, this has already been covered on p 62.

7: RENAL AND URINARY TRACT TUBERCULOSIS

7.1 How it arises

Renal tuberculosis is due to spread in the blood from the primary infection. Disease usually develops late, 5–15 years after the first infection. It seems not to be a common form of tuberculosis, even in countries with high prevalence of tuberculosis. It is rare in children. It is usually only on one side.

The disease usually starts in the outer part of the kidney (cortex). As it spreads it destroys kidney tissue and forms a cavity. If inflammatory material obstructs the junction between the kidney and the ureter, the back pressure may lead to widespread destruction of the kidney. Infection spreads to the ureter (which may become obstructed). It spreads also to the bladder (where ulcers may form), and then on to prostate, seminal vesicles and epididymis.

7.2 How it may show in the patient (clinical features)

1. **Frequency** of passing urine.
2. **Pain on passing urine.**
3. **Pain in the loin**; usually dull, sometimes acute (renal colic).
4. **Blood in urine**. If the disease is mainly in the kidney, with little bladder infection, blood in the urine may be the only symptom. Remember a renal tumour is another possible cause. In some countries bilharziasis is a common cause.
5. Swelling of the **epididymis** (p 127).
6. **Pus in the urine**. Culture for non-tuberculous bacteria will be nega-

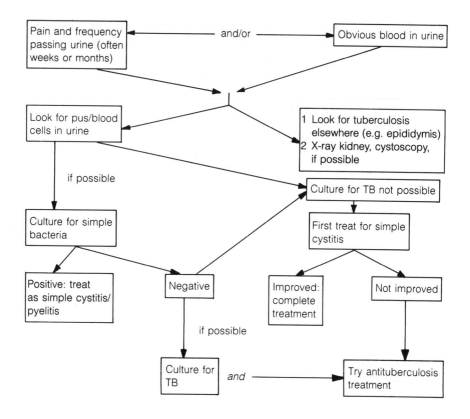

Figure 31   Flow chart: *diagnosing urinary tuberculosis*

tive. **If a patient has frequency and pain on passing urine, pus in the urine but a negative culture, tuberculosis is the most common cause.**

7.   **Loin abscess** in advanced cases.

7.3   How to diagnose it

The flow chart in Figure 31 may help you in making the diagnosis:
   Note the following points:

1.   **Urine**: examine for pus and TB. Smear examination can be misleading. Harmless non-tuberculous acid-fast bacteria are common in the urine. Don't rely on this for diagnosis unless other evidence points to tuberculosis. Culture for TB, if possible, is the reliable method but of course takes some weeks.
2.   **X-ray of kidney**: the best method is the intravenous pyelogram which can be very helpful if it is available.

3. **Clinical examination of epididymis and testes** can be very useful (p 127). Examine the prostate **per rectum**. Instead of a smooth surface you may be able to feel craggy areas on one or both sides.
5. **X-ray chest**: usually there is no abnormality.
6. **Tuberculin test**: not usually helpful.
7. **Blood urea** (if available) will tell you whether the other kidney is functioning normally.

Where few investigations are possible: If you cannot culture the urine or do X-rays you will have to decide on clinical grounds whether to treat. Frequency and pain on passing water will usually have **come on gradually**. They will have been present for weeks or months before you see the patient. As acute cystitis usually starts suddenly it soon brings the patient for help.

Then look carefully for evidence of tuberculosis elsewhere, especially in the epididymis (p 127).

If in doubt, give standard treatment for a simple cystitis. If the patient does not improve you should try anti-tuberculosis chemotherapy (p 165). Symptoms will usually start improving within 10 days.

Management is described on p 175.

A CASE OF GENITO-URINARY TUBERCULOSIS

Mr Mwasa, aged 44, came to a health post in a rural area. He had had **pain on passing urine** for about 3 months. He had to **pass urine frequently**. He had to get up 5 or 6 times during the night. He thought that sometimes there might have been **blood** in his urine. He did not feel well and he thought he had lost weight.

The Health Assistant gave him a **simple antibiotic for cystitis**. After a week there was no improvement. So he referred the patient to the small District Hospital half a day's walk away. The doctor there examined the patient carefully. He found an irregular, craggy, painless swelling in the upper part of the right epididymis. He did a rectal examination and felt an irregular swelling in the right lobe of the prostate.

The doctor sent the **urine** for examination. There were many pus cells and red cells in the deposit. Acid-fast bacilli were also present. There were no bilharzial eggs: bilharzia was quite common in that area. Because of what the doctor had found in the epididymis and prostate, and the patient's history, he thought that this was a **tuberculous cystitis**, probably with renal disease also. The acid-fast bacilli partly confirmed this. But he knew that non-tuberculous acid-fast bacilli could be found in the urine, so that only partly confirmed the diagnosis. There were **no facilities for culture or for intravenous pyelograms** in this small hospital. The nearest hospital where this could be done was several days' journey away. The patient was unwilling to make the journey.

As the patient was not very ill and had a fairly short history, the doctor decided it was best to treat him with **anti-tuberculosis chemotherapy** and watch him carefully. But to be on the safe side he checked 2 further specimens for bilharzia eggs. Both were negative.

Mr Mwasa **rapidly improved with treatment**. His urinary symptoms disappeared in 2–3 weeks. His appetite increased and he gained weight. The doctor had carefully and kindly explained about the disease and the treatment. He had told the patient and his family how important it was to go on with the treatment for the full period, even if he might lose his symptoms and feel well after a few weeks. So Mr Mwasa came back regularly and finished his treatment.

Comment: Of course it would have been safer to have had an intravenous pyelogram and to check on whether the ureter was obstructed. This was not possible. The patient obviously did very well. Even if the kidney had been damaged by an obstruction of the ureter, usually only one kidney is diseased. The other kidney, if normal, could function normally and prevent renal failure.

8: TUBERCULOSIS OF FEMALE GENITAL TRACT

8.1 How it arises

Genital tuberculosis in the female arises as a result of blood spread after primary infection. It affects the endometrium and fallopian tubes.

8.2 How it shows in the patient

1. **Infertility** is the commonest reason for seeking help. The diagnosis is often made as a result of routine investigation for infertility. This should always include looking for signs of tuberculosis.
2. **Lower abdominal or pelvic pain, malaise**, disturbance of **rhythm of menstruation** (including amenorrhoea or bleeding), postmenopausal bleeding.
3. Progression to **abscess formation** of the fallopian tube. Sometimes with large **abdominal masses**.
4. **Ectopic pregnancy**.

8.3 Investigations

1. Pelvic examination: masses, which may be small or large, may be felt over the fallopian tube area.
2. X-ray of genital tract, if this is possible.

8.4   Treatment

Patients improve very well with chemotherapy (p 165). Large masses may just fade away. Surgery for these is unnecessary.

Although the disease is always arrested if chemotherapy is taken properly, damage to the fallopian tube may obstruct its very small lumen. So the patient may remain infertile. Because the ovum may not be able to get through the narrowed tube **ectopic pregnancy** (in the tube, not the uterus) may occur later. Skilled surgical treatment of the blocked tube, if available, can sometimes restore fertility.

9: TUBERCULOSIS OF MALE GENITAL TRACT

9.1   How it arises

The prostate, seminal vesicles and epididymis are involved separately or together. Infection may come from the blood stream or from the kidney through the urinary tract (p 123).

9.2   How it shows in the patient (clinical features)

Most often the patient comes up complaining of something wrong with one of his 'testes'. In fact this is usually the epididymis, not the testis itself. The **epididymis** enlarges and becomes hard and craggy, usually starting at its upper pole. It is usually only slightly tender. An acute non-tuberculous epididymitis is usually very tender and painful. The lesion in the epididymis may break down into an **abscess**, involve the skin and result in a **sinus**. You should also examine the **seminal vesicles** by the rectum. The **prostate** may feel craggy and you may be able to feel the seminal vesicles on each side, above and lateral to the prostate. If you can feel them they are probably abnormal.

In 40 per cent of cases the patient will also have the symptoms and signs of **urinary tuberculosis**.

9.3   Investigations

1. Urine etc. for evidence of tuberculosis (p 124).
2. X-ray of kidney if this is possible (p 124).
3. Tuberculin test is rarely helpful.

9.4   Diagnosis

1. Acute epididymitis: fever, chills, acute pain locally.
2. Tumour: usually smooth and hard. The craggy mass of tuberculosis is usually typical.

9.5 Treatment

Treatment with chemotherapy is normally completely successful if fully taken (see p 165).

Surgical treatment is only needed if tumour is suspected.

10: INTESTINAL/PERITONEAL TUBERCULOSIS

10.1 How it arises

There are three forms of abdominal tuberculosis: primary, secondary and hyperplastic ileo-caecal tuberculosis. Clinically, the primary and secondary forms may be very similar.

1. The **primary focus** has been described on p 30. Formerly in Europe it was usually caused by bovine TB through infection from cows' milk. The primary lesion was presumably in the bowel wall but it was the mesenteric (abdominal) lymph nodes, and spread from them, which caused most of the symptoms. In some cases the disease arises from bloodborne spread through the lymph nodes or the peritoneum. This may be more common in Asia and Africa where bovine disease is often thought to be rare, though in many countries we still do not have sufficient information: see p 7. The **lymph nodes** enlarge and get matted together. If they rupture, infection spreads into the peritoneal cavity and effusion occurs (**ascites**). The adhesion of nodes to bowel may cause **obstruction**. Communications (**fistulae**) may occur between the bowel and bladder or bowel and abdominal wall.
2. In the **secondary form** patients with pulmonary tuberculosis swallow their sputum. The TB in the sputum infect the wall of the intestine (usually the ileum) and cause **ulceration**. **Fistulae** may occur as described above. Infection may spread into the abdominal cavity and cause **ascites**.
3. **Hyperplastic ileo-caecal tuberculosis** is a rare form of the disease. It occurs in the region of the ileo-caecal valve.

10.2 How it shows in the patient (clinical features)

There may be the following symptoms or signs:

1. **Loss of weight,** loss of **appetite**: very common.
2. **Abdominal pain** (often vague); **fever; night sweats; diarrhoea;** loss of **menstrual periods**.
3. **Abdominal mass** or masses (often rather soft to feel). There is often also fluid in the abdomen (**ascites**). Sometimes there is so much fluid

that you cannot feel any mass, so that the main sign is ascites. In **hyperplastic ileo-caecal tuberculosis** there may be **pain** and a **mass** to be felt in the right lower abdomen. There may be no signs elsewhere. This can be confused with a cancer of the bowel.

4. Attacks of **intestinal obstruction** with acute pain and distension of the abdomen.
5. **Cough** and **sputum** if the bowel disease is caused by swallowing the sputum from pulmonary tuberculosis (secondary form).

10.3   Diagnosis

SUSPECT THE POSSIBILITY OF ABDOMINAL TUBERCULOSIS IN ANY PATIENT WHO IS LOSING WEIGHT, HAS FEVER, AND HAS VAGUE ABDOMINAL PAIN. BE EVEN MORE SUSPICIOUS IF THERE IS AN ABDOMINAL MASS OR FLUID IN THE ABDOMEN.

You will usually have to make the diagnosis on clinical grounds. But sometimes additional help may be obtained from:

1. **X-ray** examination of the bowel.
2. **Biopsy of lymph node or peritoneum** at operation or laparoscopy (insertion of lighted tube into the abdomen).
3. **Culture** of material from aspiration of liquid from the abdominal cavity or from pus from sinuses.

Sometimes a patient has only **recurrent vague abdominal pain**. There may be no obvious fluid or masses to be felt. There may be little fever. If it is not possible to carry out any of the above investigations it is worth while **trying the effect of chemotherapy**. If the disease is tuberculosis the patient soon loses the symptoms and begins to improve.

10.4   Treatment

Chemotherapy is usually highly effective (p 165). Even large masses fade away. Occasionally healed disease leaves adhesions between loops of intestine, or scarring. These sometimes later cause mechanical obstruction of the bowel which may need surgery. If there is a large amount of fluid you may have to aspirate it. It may be useful then to give prednisolone as well as chemotherapy (p 188), if this is available.

10.5   Fistula-in-ano

This is a fistula or sinus in the region of the anus. It may complicate abdominal tuberculosis, but may be the only obvious lesion. In high prevalence countries tuberculosis is the commonest cause. But it can occur with ulcerative colitis, Crohn's disease and other conditions. When due to tuberculosis, it improves rapidly with chemotherapy.

11: TUBERCULOSIS OF THE EYE

This may occur at any age. The different types have been described in the section on children's tuberculosis, p 69.

12: ADRENAL TUBERCULOSIS

12.1   General comments

In countries where tuberculosis is common it may cause half the cases of adrenal insufficiency (**Addison's disease**). In tuberculosis the TB reach the adrenals through the blood stream.

The main symptoms are severe **tiredness** and general **weakness**. There is often recurrent **vomiting** and **diarrhoea**. A common and valuable clue to diagnosis is **pigmentation** of the skin. This occurs particularly over pressure areas e.g. elbows or lower thoracic spine. It also occurs in **patches inside the mouth**: this is particularly valuable in races with naturally pigmented skin. The **blood pressure** is low. Sometimes the **tuberculin test** may be helpful.

The **serum sodium** is often below normal, if you can test it. This is due to repeated vomiting and/or diarrhoea. High plasma potassium is even more frequent. This is due to lack of aldosterone.

X-ray of the abdomen (if you can get it) shows calcification in the region of the adrenals in about 20 per cent of cases. Tuberculous adrenal glands are usually enlarged, but this can only be shown by ultrasound or tomography which is often not available.

AIDS may produce similar symptoms. Remember the possibility of Addison's disease as you can treat this effectively. **Remember to look for patches of pigment in the mouth**.

12.2   Treatment

The tuberculosis can be cured with chemotherapy (p 165). But replacement of the missing hormones is always necessary. You must send the patient to an appropriate hospital specialist.

13: CUTANEOUS (SKIN) AND SUBCUTANEOUS (ABSCESSES) TUBERCULOSIS

Skin tuberculosis is not very common but the diagnosis is often missed. If you make the right diagnosis on a skin condition it may also help you to find tuberculosis somewhere else in the body.

.There are a number of different types of skin conditions due to tuberculosis.

13.1   Primary lesions

See p 72.

13.2   Erythema nodosum

This is a type of **hypersensitivity to tuberculin**. Usually, but not always, it occurs at the same time as the primary infection. It appears to be much rarer in patients with dark skins than in whites. Maybe this is because the skin lesions are less obvious on dark skins. An Indian physician informs us that, after learning to recognise erythema nodosm in Europe, he has frequently diagnosed it in association with tuberculosis in India. It is not only due to tuberculosis. **Other causes** include streptococcal infection, drugs, sarcoidosis, leprosy, histoplasmosis and coccidioidomycosis.

It is rare before age 7 and **commoner in females** at all ages. There is often preliminary **fever** which may be high in young women. Women may also have pain in the larger **joints**, which may be hot and tender as in rheumatic fever.

The most obvious finding is tender, dusky red, slightly nodular **lesions on the front of the legs** below the knee. They feel deep to the skin rather than in it. They are 5–20 mm in diameter and with ill-defined margins. They may run together to become confluent, usually above the ankles. This produces a firm, tender, dusky red area. Recurrent crops of lesions may occur over weeks.

If you suspect erythema nodosum look carefully for evidence of tuberculosis, or one of the other causes given above. The tuberculin test is usually very strongly positive. There may be severe skin, or even general reaction with fever, to the normal dose of tuberculin. Give a tenth of the normal dose (p 201) first. If there is no reaction then give the normal dose. If there is tuberculosis, the erythema nodosum usually improves very rapidly with treatment.

13.3 Miliary lesions

These are rare but may become more common in patients with HIV infection and tuberculosis. They may or may not be associated with generalised miliary tuberculosis (p 107). There are three forms:

1. multiple small copper coloured spots,
2. multiple papules which break down in the middle and form pustules,
3. multiple subcutaneous abscesses on the arms and legs, the chest wall or the buttocks: perianal abscesses (abscesses near the anus) may also occur.

13.4 Verrucous tuberculosis

These lesions occur in patients with a good deal of immunity to tuberculosis. They are particularly seen in health professionals. 'Warty' lesions appear on exposed parts of the body. Regional lymph nodes are not enlarged.

13.5 Ulcers of mouth, nose and anus

These usually occur in people with advanced tuberculosis. They may be painful.

13.6 Scrofuloderma

This results from direct invasion and breakdown of the skin from an underlying tuberculous lesion, usually a lymph node – sometimes bone or epididymis. Sinuses usually develop and leave a scar when they heal.

13.7 Lupus vulgaris

This usually affects the head and neck. Commonly it occurs over the bridge of the nose and on to the cheeks. Jelly-like nodules appear. These sometimes ulcerate. They may cause extensive scarring and destruction of the face. TB are rarely seen but the tuberculin test is usually positive. It is usually very chronic. The diagnosis may be missed for many years.

13.8 Tuberculides

These are slightly painful, slightly raised, bluish red local rounded thickenings of the skin. They appear mainly on the back of the calf. The tuberculin test is almost always positive. Such lesions are not always caused by tuberculosis. But if you can be sure that it is not due to tuberculosis you will often not be able to find the true cause.

13.9   Treatment

All skin and subcutaneous lesions do very well with anti-tuberculosis chemotherapy.

In countries with high prevalence of tuberculosis, DO REMEMBER THE POSSIBILITY OF TUBERCULOSIS WHENEVER YOU SEE A CHRONIC PAINLESS SKIN CONDITION. If you suspect the skin diagnosis, look for tuberculous lesions elsewhere in the patient.

5
Tuberculosis, HIV (Human Immunodeficiency Virus) Infection and AIDS (Acquired ImmunoDeficiency Syndrome)

The rapid increase of HIV infection in many parts of the world is causing **great problems in the diagnosis and treatment of tuberculosis**. It is also causing **great problems in tuberculosis control**. In 1995 worldwide there were about 17 million HIV-infected cases. An estimated 6 million adult and paediatric AIDS cases have occurred since the HIV pandemic began. About a third of people infected with HIV were also infected with TB. Of these 70 per cent were in Africa, 20 per cent in Asia and 8 per cent in Latin America. By the year 2000 WHO expects that 40 per cent of all TB patients in Africa will also be HIV-infected, 18 per cent in South East Asia and 15 per cent in Latin America.

For the problem of **HIV and tuberculosis in children** see p 82.

1: BACKGROUND

1.1 HIV and AIDS

AIDS is due to the **Human Immunodeficiency Virus (HIV)**. This virus seems to have first appeared in the world in the 1970s. Researchers have identified two types of HIV. HIV-1 is the predominant type worldwide and HIV-2 occurs most commonly in West Africa. The virus gradually destroys the body's defensive cells. So **the body cannot defend itself against infection**. In countries with high prevalence of tuberculosis, 30–60 per cent of adults have been infected **with TB**. Most people's defences prevent the TB causing **disease**. But if their defences have been damaged by HIV the TB may no longer be kept under control. They may multiply and cause disease. In the same way, people with HIV infection, even if not yet ill, may not be able to resist new infection with TB from other patients with a positive sputum. So there are likely to be many

Note: Much of this chapter is based, with permission, on the WHO booklet *TB/HIV. A Clinical Manual*: see reference at end of chapter.

more cases of tuberculosis in countries where there is increasing HIV infection. **In some sub-Saharan African countries 20–70 per cent of patients with tuberculosis have been shown to be HIV positive**.

1.2   The HIV virus

The **HIV virus** can be **spread** in different ways:

1. By **heterosexual** activity between man and woman.
2. By **homosexual** activity, man to man.
3. Through **blood** by:
    a) Blood transfusion with blood untested for HIV. (In countries where many people are becoming infected with HIV, even screened blood can be dangerous. There may be virus in the blood before antibodies can be detected.)
    b) Use of needles which have not been properly sterilised. This is common in **drug abusers**.
4. From mother to child: **congenital transmission**. Also by breast feeding: see p 83. About one-third of children born to HIV-infected mothers are also HIV-infected.

APART FROM SEXUAL ACTIVITY OR BLOOD CONTAMINATION THERE IS NO PERSON-TO-PERSON RISK. It is NOT DANGEROUS to care for AIDS or HIV-infected patients as long as you are careful about needles and blood. (However health staff who are known to be HIV-infected, even if healthy, should not care for patients with TB. They have a much greater risk than normal people of being infected with TB and later developing disease.)

1.3   Geographical spread

The amount of HIV infection in the sexually active population is already 10–25 per cent in some cities in sub-Saharan Africa and parts of Latin America, especially the Caribbean. It is increasing in North America, Europe and Australasia. It is rapidly increasing in South East Asia.

In North America, with a low prevalence of infection with TB, AIDS patients often develop infection with opportunistic mycobacteria (p 199), not TB. Nevertheless there have been important outbreaks of TB among the HIV-infected. Some have been with multiple resistant bacilli. In countries with a high prevalence of tuberculosis, it is tuberculosis that develops in HIV-infected patients.

There is a long period, often several years, between infection with the HIV virus and developing AIDS. This period is shorter in children under five and in patients aged over forty. During this 'incubation period' the patient may feel quite well (though he/she remains infectious). **The development of tuberculosis is often the first sign that he/she has HIV**

infection. In about 50 per cent of patients with HIV and tuberculosis there is no other evidence of HIV infection. The only way to make the diagnosis is to do an HIV test. There is evidence that tuberculosis in an HIV-infected patient may speed the development of full clinical AIDS. In sub-Saharan Africa and now in Asia, heterosexual spread of AIDS is the commonest. So tuberculosis may complicate HIV in both sexes.

1.4 Drugs

At present (1997) there is **no effective vaccine** for HIV. The newer drugs, especially if given in combination, do delay the onset and progress of AIDS but are still very expensive: see paragraph 8, p 145.

1.5 Diagnosis and testing

You yourself are likely to see the patient only when he comes with symptoms and signs of tuberculosis or other infection. But often the symptoms and signs are unusual (see below). You can only be certain whether he has underlying HIV infection by doing a blood test for **HIV antibodies**. Because the outlook of the diagnosis is so bad, the rule in your country is probably that **you must ask the patient's permission to do this test**. You must also counsel him (or her) carefully and kindly as to why the test is necessary and what the result (positive or negative) may mean to him/her: see paragraph 6 below.

This also means you must **counsel him/her carefully and kindly when you get the result, whether it is positive or negative** (paragraph 6 below).

The HIV antibody test is the only certain way of making the diagnosis. But this may not be possible where you are working. In that case you will have to decide by considering all the clinical facts in the patient's case.

2: EFFECT OF HIV ON CONTROL PROGRAMMES

2.1 Disease prevalence

In countries with high TB prevalence, HIV infection is much the most important factor making a person liable to get clinical TB. Among people already infected with TB (as shown by being tuberculin positive) their **lifetime risk of clinical TB** is about 50 per cent if they have been infected with HIV. This compares with a 5–10 per cent risk if they are HIV negative. The result is a **great increase of TB cases** where and when the HIV rate becomes high. This puts a major strain on services.

2.2   Sputum testing

Sputum positivity is less common in TB/HIV. Symptoms of HIV and TB are often similar. The result can be that health workers may make a diagnosis of sputum-negative TB and give TB treatment when the patient's symptoms are not due to TB. So there may be gross overuse of anti-TB drugs. This wastes resources without helping patients.

2.3   Drug reactions

Drug reactions are much more common in TB/HIV. This may increase the default rate from treatment.

2.4   Separation of patients

In hospitals definite TB patients and those who might prove to have TB must be **kept separate** from HIV patients as these are so easily infected. And if infected they are more likely to develop TB disease.

2.5   HIV-positive staff

For the same reason serum **HIV-positive staff** must not look after TB patients.

2.6   Needles

Great care must be taken in using **needles**. For this reason streptomycin is no longer used for tuberculosis in many countries with high HIV prevalence. (For full precautions see Appendix p 151.)

3: HOW TUBERCULOSIS WITH HIV INFECTION SHOWS CLINICALLY

The following are differences from the usual ways tuberculosis shows in patients without HIV infection:

1. **Extra-pulmonary disease**, especially in the lymph nodes, is more common. There is often **general** lymph node enlargement, which is rare in other forms of tuberculosis.
2. **Miliary disease** is common. TB may be isolated from blood culture (which never occurs in ordinary tuberculosis).
3. **X-ray.** In the early stages of HIV infection with pulmonary TB there is often little difference in the X-ray from the usual appearances. In

the later stages there are often **large mediastinal lymph node masses**. There is often **lower lobe disease**. The shadow may be only in the lower lobe and not very extensive. **Cavitation may be less frequent**. **Pleural and pericardial effusions** are more common. The shadows in the lung may **change rapidly**.

4. Tuberculosis may occur at **unusual sites**, e.g. tuberculomas of the brain (p 58), abcesses of the chest wall (p 73) or elsewhere.
5. **Sputum smears may be negative** despite considerable changes in the chest X-ray.
6. **The tuberculin test is often negative**.
7. **Fever and weight loss** are **more** common in HIV-positive tuberculosis than in HIV-negative. On the other hand **cough and blood spitting** are **less** common.

In a patient with tuberculosis, suspect the possibility of accompanying HIV infection if there is:

- general lymph node enlargement. In late stages of HIV the nodes may be tender and painful, as in acute infection
- candida infection (painful white patches of fungus in the mouth)
- chronic diarrhoea for more than a month
- herpes zoster (shingles)
- Kaposi's sarcoma: look for small red vascular nodules on the skin, and particularly on the palate
- generalised itchy dermatitis
- chronic increasing or generalised herpes simplex
- burning feeling in the feet (due to neuropathy)
- persistent painful ulceration of genitalia.

4: NOTE ON WHO CASE DEFINITIONS FOR AIDS

We give these for reference. They may be useful to you for your general clinical work as well as in your tuberculosis work. The definitions are as follows:

4.1 Where HIV testing is not available

You may diagnose AIDS if there are at least two of the following major signs and at least one minor sign:

Major signs

- weight loss more than 10 per cent of body weight
- chronic diarrhoea for more than one month
- prolonged fever for more than one month

Minor signs

- persistent cough for more than one month
- generalised pruritic (itchy) dermatitis
- history of herpes zoster (shingles)
- candida infection (painful white patches of fungus in the mouth)
- chronic increasing or generalised herpes simplex
- generalised enlargement of lymph nodes

Note that weight loss, prolonged fever and persistent cough can be due to tuberculosis. To decide whether a patient has tuberculosis or AIDS the other signs are therefore more important (see list in paragraph 3 above). If you have proved that the patient has tuberculosis, e.g. by a positive sputum, these other signs may show you that he/she also has HIV.

4.2 Where HIV testing is available

You can diagnose AIDS if there is a positive HIV test and one or more of the following:

- weight loss greater than 10 per cent of body weight, or cachexia (advanced state of illness with wasting and weakness) with diarrhoea or fever or both, for at least one month and not known to be due to some other disease
- cryptococcal meningitis
- tuberculosis (pulmonary or non-pulmonary)
- Kaposi's sarcoma
- neurological weakness which prevents independent daily activities, not known to be due to another disease
- oesophageal candidiasis (fungus infection)
- life-threatening or recurrent pneumonia
- invasive cervical cancer.

4.3 Children (see also p 82)

4.3.1 Where HIV testing not available. You can diagnose AIDS if there are at least two major and two minor signs as follows (if there is no other known cause of immunosuppression).

Major signs

- weight loss or abnormally slow growth
- chronic diarrhoea (for more than one month)
- prolonged fever (for more than one month)

Minor signs

- generalised lymph node enlargement

- mouth candidiasis (fungal infection)
- recurrent common infections, e.g. ear infections, sore throats
- persistent cough
- generalised rash

4.3.2 *Where HIV testing is available.* The case definition is complex as an infant may inherit the mother's HIV antibodies without inheriting the virus. A positive test indicates that there may or may not be viral infection. So clinical signs, as above, are the most important indication of disease.

Inherited antibodies gradually disappear if there is no viral infection. A positive test in a child aged 2 years or more indicates infection.

5: NON-TUBERCULOUS COMPLICATIONS OF HIV INFECTION

You need to know about these. You may have to distinguish them from tuberculosis. Or they may occur in a patient in addition to tuberculosis. Or they may occur later on when your treatment has controlled the patient's tuberculosis. They are:

5.1 Early HIV illness

Most patients remain well after infection for months or years. The HIV only shows itself when the patient develops a complication, notably tuberculosis. But a few patients may develop an illness when their serum becomes positive for HIV, usually 6 weeks to 3 months after infection. The illness is often like 'glandular fever' (infectious mononucleosis): fever, rash, joint pains and enlarged lymph nodes. In severe cases there may be in addition aseptic meningitis, encephalitis (brain inflammation), myelitis (spinal cord inflammation) or peripheral nerve inflammation. These usually clear up without specific treatment.

5.2 Kaposi's sarcoma

Diagnosis is easy if you find small red vascular nodules on the skin. These may be less obvious in dark skins. Look particularly at the palate where they may be more obvious.

Lesions in the lung or pleura are more difficult to diagnose. They are more likely to be confused with tuberculosis. The patient usually has cough, fever and breathlessness. X-ray, if available, may show diffuse nodules and/or pleural effusion. The effusion is usually bloodstained. If there is any doubt, treat the treatable diagnosis, i.e. tuberculosis.

5.3　*Pneumocystis carinii* pneumonia (PCP)

This is less common in Africa than elsewhere. The patient usually has dry cough and increasing breathlessness. In tuberculosis he is more likely to have purulent or bloodstained sputum and chest pain. In PCP the X-ray may be normal or show diffuse interstitial shadowing in both lungs. Definite diagnosis depends on finding the cysts in the sputum or bronchial lavage but you may not have facilities for this.

If a patient with well treated and controlled tuberculosis becomes increasingly breathless, first check that there is no increasing pneumonia. Also check that he does not have cardiac failure, asthma or anaemia. If you find none of these, the explanation may well be PCP infection. If you cannot test for this, try giving high dose co-trimoxazole (3–4 tablets 4 times daily) together with a tapering course of prednisolone (if available). (Advice from Professor A.D. Harries).

5.4　Pulmonary cryptococcosis

This may look like tuberculosis. Definite diagnosis depends on finding fungal spores in the sputum.

5.5　Nocardiasis

This may look very like tuberculosis on the X-ray and the organism may stain weakly acid fast. Abscesses in brain or soft tissue should make you think of this possibility. Definite diagnosis depends on finding beaded and branching Gram-positive rods in a sputum smear. But of course look for TB first!

6: HIV TESTING AND COUNSELLING

6.1　HIV testing

A positive HIV serum test is proof of the diagnosis. This may not be possible where you work: you will have to make the diagnosis clinically (see above).

If the test is available consider offering it to your tuberculosis patients. Many will know that HIV is often associated. Testing may have the following advantages for the patient:

1. A definite negative test will relieve his anxiety: but counsel him/her about future risks and their avoidance, e.g. condom use.
2. Better diagnosis and management of other HIV-related illnesses.
3. Avoidance of drugs, especially thioacetazone, with high risk of dangerous side-effects.
4. If positive, condom use to avoid infecting others.

6.2 Laboratory testing

The standard laboratory test is the ELISA (Enzyme-Linked ImmunoSorbent Assay) on serum. If positive, it is safer to repeat it and confirm. If the second test is negative, do two more tests to be sure the positive was not an error. In poorer countries it may only be possible to do one test and find it either negative or positive.

6.3 Pre-test counselling (see also p 85)

Only test after counselling the patient on the advantages. Find out what he/she knows about HIV. Make sure he/she understands what a positive test will mean for his/her life. This covers both health and social/family aspects. There is probably a standard outline designed for the culture of the area where you work. There are probably local health workers, social workers or volunteers trained to counsel.

6.4 Post-test counselling

Counselling and support is obviously vital if the test proves positive. Make sure he/she knows that you will cure his tuberculosis in spite of the HIV. Work with any local organisation for the counselling and support of HIV patients. Make sure the following are discussed:

- general health: diet, rest, exercise, avoiding infections (especially sexual)
- when to seek help for symptoms of other HIV-related illnesses
- possible side-effects of anti-tuberculosis drugs
- safe sexual behaviour with partners (condoms)
- avoid blood or organ donation
- patient's reaction to test result
- emotional and psychological support
- how to tell family, friends, lovers
- counselling partners
- social implications, e.g. employment, life insurance
- referral to local support services and groups when available.

7: TREATMENT OF TUBERCULOSIS

7.1   Short-course treatment

Modern short-course treatment of tuberculosis in an HIV-positive patient is as effective as in HIV-negative patients. The sputum becomes negative just as quickly. Relapse rates are no higher. Weight gain may be somewhat less than in HIV-negative patients. But with former long term 'standard' treatment, not including rifampicin, treatment was less successful and relapse much commoner. Some of the relapse may have been due to reinfection because of the patient's lowered defences from HIV.

7.2   Mortality

Nevertheless there is a **higher mortality** in HIV infected patients. Much of this is due to other complications of HIV infection (see below). But some deaths seem directly due to tuberculosis.

7.3   Prognosis

The long term prognosis is therefore poor, as in all HIV patients. But treatment of the patient's tuberculosis does usually give him/her a longer period of improved health and is well worth doing. Moreover treatment stops the spread of tuberculosis to others. Unfortunately tuberculosis seems to speed up the progress of the HIV illness.

7.4   Side-effects

Side-effects of drugs are commoner in HIV-positive patients. In particular thioacetazone is liable to cause severe skin reactions (p 184, 186). These may be fatal in up to 25 per cent of cases. Tell the patient to stop treatment if he gets itching and report at once. This can prevent a severe reaction. If a patient develops a reaction to thiaoacetazone NEVER USE IT AGAIN. Use ethambutol instead. (For details of management see p 186). Some countries with high prevalence of HIV no longer use thioacetazone.

7.5   Streptomycin

Streptomycin has to be given by injection. This carries a risk of spreading HIV from blood contamination. In countries with a high prevalence of HIV and which cannot afford a new syringe for each patient it is better to use ethambutol instead of streptomycin.

8: TREATMENT OF HIV INFECTION

Newer drugs (e.g. zidovudine, lamivudine, nelfinavir, ritonavir, loviride) given to HIV infected patients do delay the onset and progress of AIDS. They seem to be most effective if given in combination, perhaps with three drugs together. At present the drugs are much too expensive for a national programme in poorer countries. It is still too soon to talk about a 'cure' but the situation is getting more hopeful. Watch out for further news as research and clinical trials develop. As we write, WHO is exploring possible pilot schemes to find how best to use these drugs in poorer countries.

For counselling patients positive for HIV see paragraph 6.4 above.

Your patients with TB/HIV may develop **other infections and complications**. We briefly outline below how to manage the commoner ones. For more details see references at the end of this chapter.

9: TREATMENT OF OTHER COMPLICATIONS OF HIV INFECTION

9.1 Sexually transmitted diseases (STDs)

In countries where most HIV is spread heterosexually, a patient with HIV is liable also to other STDs. Indeed a patient with STD has a higher risk of HIV infection if he/she is exposed to the virus.

You may not have the resources to make an accurate diagnosis of STD. So WHO has developed 'syndrome management'. Each 'syndrome' is a group of symptoms and signs. The treatment recommended for each syndrome will cure most patients with that syndrome. The syndromes and the plan of treatment for each are as shown in Table 7.

Treat each of the diseases under 'Plan of Treatment' in Table 7, as described in Table 8.

Important notes (a) The following tables are shortened versions of those in the WHO TB/HIV book. We have included fewer alternative treatments. For more detail consult the WHO book. (b) Do not use tetracycline in pregnant patients or children: it damages the teeth of the infant or child.

Table 7 *STD syndromes and management*

Sex	Syndrome	Plan of treatment
Men	Urethral discharge	Treat for gonorrhoea and chlamydia
Women	Cervicitis	Treat for uncomplicated gonorrhoea and chlamydia
	Vaginitis	Treat for candidiasis and *Trichomonas vaginalis*/bacterial vaginosis
	Vaginal discharge	Treat for cervicitis and vaginitis
Men and women	Genital ulcers	Treat for syphilis and chancroid
	Inguinal bubo (enlarged tender lymph nodes)	
	• with ulcers	Treat for syphilis and chancroid
	• without ulcers	Treat for lymphogranuloma venereum

Table 8 *STD treatment*

STD	Treatments
Gonorrhoea (uncomplicated)	Trimethoprim (80 mg)/sulfamethoxazole (400 mg) (TMP–SMX): 10 tablets orally as a single dose **OR** If you can use a separate disposable syringe and needle for each patient: gentamicin 240 mg by intramuscular (IM) injection.
Chlamydia	Tetracycline 500 mg orally × 4 daily for 7 days **OR** Erythromycin 500 mg × 4 daily for 7 days (especially for pregnant women)
Primary syphilis (chancre)	Tetracycline 500 mg orally × 4 daily for 15 days **OR** If you can give it safely (see above): benzathine penicillin G 2.4 million Units by IM injection at a single session (often split into 2 doses at separate sites)
Chancroid	Erythromycin 500 mg × 3 daily for 7 days **OR** TMP–SMX (see above) 2 tablets orally × 2 daily for 7 days
Lymphogranuloma venereum	Tetracycline 500 mg orally × 4 daily for 14 days **OR** Erythromycin 500 mg in a single dose daily for 14 days
Candidiasis	Nystatin 100,000 Units intra-vaginally once daily for 14 days
Trichomonas vaginalis	Metronidazole 2 g orally as a single dose
Bacterial vaginosis	Metronidazole 2 g orally as a single dose

9.2   Skin and mouth problems

The treatment for the various problems is summarised in Table 9.

Table 9   *Treatment of skin and mouth problems*

Diagnosis	Treatment
Skin problems	
Virus infections (Note: Aciclovir may not be affordable in low income countries)	
Herpes simplex (oral and genital)	Local lesion care ± (if severe): Aciclovir 200 mg orally × 5 daily until healed
Varicella zoster ('Herpes zoster')	Local lesion care ±: Aciclovir 800 mg orally × 5 daily for at least 7 days
Anal/genital warts (human papilloma virus)	Topical 20% podophyllin × 1–2 per week until cleared
Molluscum contagiosum	Leave lesions alone **OR** Prick each lesion with a sharpened orange stick or needle and touch with phenol. (Use a new stick or needle for each patient and then discard)
Fungal infections	
Tinea (feet, body, groin)	Whitfield's ointment or Castellani's paint
Candidiasis	Local application of 1% aqueous gentian violet **OR** Nystatin ointment × 2 daily till cleared
Cutaneous cryptococcosis or histoplasmosis	Systemic antifungal drugs
Bacterial infections	
Impetigo, furunculosis	Penicillin V 500 mg orally × 4 daily for 1–2 weeks
Pyomyositis (purulent infection of muscles)	Surgical drainage + antibiotics (as for impetigo)
Other	
Papular folliculitis of skin with itching	Calamine lotion, antihistamines If very severe: corticosteroids applied locally
Seborrhoeic dermatitis	Local antifungals **OR** Local 1% hydrocortisone
Psoriasis	Coal tar in salicylate ointment × 2 daily
Scabies	Local benzyl benzoate 25%
Kaposi sarcoma	Local lesion care Radiotherapy or chemotherapy if available

Mouth problems

Candidiasis of mouth	Nystatin drops × 3 daily for 7–14 days **OR** Nystatin tablets 500,000 Units × 4 daily for 7–14 days
Angular stomatitis (inflammation of angles of lips)	Local antifungals, e.g. 1% clotrimazole
Gingivitis (gum inflammation/dental abscesses)	Oral metronidazole 400 mg × 3 daily and/or penicillin V 500 mg × 4 daily for 7 days
Aphthous stomatitis (painful mouth ulcers which are not candidiasis)	Mouth rinses with tetracycline and steroids

9.3   Gastrointestinal problems

Treatment of gastrointestinal problems is outlined in Table 10.

Table 10   *Treatment of gastrointestinal problems*

Diagnosis	Treatment
Dysphagia (painful swallowing) (usually due to candidiasis)	Nystatin 500 Units × 4 daily for 1–14 days **OR** Nystatin pessaries 100,000 Units every 4 hours for 1–14 days Prevention: Nystatin pastilles (If treatment fails, refer if possible to a gastroenterologist.)
Herpes simplex	Aciclovir 800 mg orally × 5 daily for 7–10 days
Ulcers of unknown cause	Prednisolone 10 mg × 4 daily for 2 weeks and then slowly decreased to zero
Diarrhoea Very common: often with nausea, vomiting, abdominal cramps, flatulence, weight loss and dehydration	If facilities: look for cause on microscopy and culture and give appropriate treatment In most cases you will not know the cause. Give rehydration: use oral rehydration solution or intravenous in severe cases
Persistent diarrhoea	Try TMP–SMX 2 tabs × 2 daily 7 days. If no response try metronidazole (Table 9) Symptomatic: codeine

9.4   Respiratory problems

HIV patients are liable to get pneumonia. First check that patient taking all his antituberculosis drugs. If so, symptoms may be due to bacterial infection as listed in Table 11.

Table 11   *Treatment of pneumonia due to bacterial infection*

Diagnosis	Treatment
Streptococcus pneumoniae	Penicillin V 750 mg 6-hourly **OR** TMP–SMX 960 mg 6-hourly
Haemophilus influenzae	Amoxycillin 250–500 mg 8-hourly (according to severity) **OR** TMP–SMX 960 mg 6-hourly
Staphylococcus aureus	Flucloxacillin 250–500 mg 6-hourly (according to severity) at least 30 minutes before food **OR** Chloramphenicol 500 mg 6-hourly
Pneumocystis carinii	See paragraph 5.3 p 142
Gram-negative bacilli	Chloramphenicol

9.5   Neurological problems

These may need careful clinical examination and investigation (if feasible) to make a diagnosis. It may be possible to get simple tests on blood or cerebrospinal fluid (CSF). We cannot cover the problems in detail but a few notes follow:

- **Acute confusion**: remember may be due to an infection, oxygen lack, metabolic illness.
- **Chronic behaviour change**: may be due to (untreatable) AIDS dementia etc. Treatable possibilities include syphilis, trypanosomiasis, chronic meningitis.
- **Persistent headache**: is unlikely to be only symptom/sign. Investigate fully as above.
- **Difficulty in walking**: check that no spinal tuberculosis (p 62). If negative, check for other causes of spinal cord disease: see textbooks.
- **Burning sensation in feet**: may be due to HIV and made worse by isoniazid. In TB/HIV patients give pyridoxine 10 mg daily (if available) to prevent this.

9.6   Septicaemia

Pneumococcus or *Salmonella typhimurium* are the commonest causes. If you cannot get a blood culture, try standard pneumococcal treatment first. *S. typhimurium* is often resistant to standard antibiotics: treat with chloramphenicol or ampicillin and gentamicin.

9.7   Anaemia

Anaemia may be due to multiple causes in HIV infection. Treat with iron and/or folic acid.

9.8   Thrombocytopenia

Thrombocytopenia (low platelet count) may be due to HIV or drug reaction. If there is bleeding use high dose steroids.

10: PREVENTIVE TREATMENT WITH ISONIAZID

This is used in HIV patients with no evidence of clinical tuberculosis. It presents a number of problems: see Appendix C p 197.

11: BCG VACCINATION

See p 86.

12: CONCLUSIONS

1. With modern short-term treatment you can cure tuberculosis in HIV patients. On average you can give the patient an extra 2 years of life.
2. By giving good treatment to TB/HIV you prevent the spread of TB infection. This is particularly important when there are many HIV positive people; these have poor defences against the disease
3. Unfortunately tuberculosis speeds up the progress of HIV disease.
4. Therefore your TB/HIV patients may develop other common complications of HIV. We have briefly outlined some of these. We have also listed some of the recommended treatments for them. For further detail see the references below.

References

Harries A.D., Maher D. *TB/HIV. A Clinical Manual*. Geneva: WHO, 1996.

WHO Global Programme on AIDS. *Counselling for HIV/AIDS: a key to caring*. Geneva: WHO, 1995.

WHO Global Programme on AIDS. *AIDS Homecare Handbook*. Geneva: WHO, 1993.

WHO Global Programme on AIDS. *Management of Sexually Transmitted Diseases*. Geneva: WHO, 1994.

APPENDIX ON PROTECTION OF HEALTH STAFF FROM INFECTION BY HIV

1. If taking blood wear gloves. Afterwards put needle and syringe into special 'Sharp Box'. Put gloves and swabs into leak-proof plastic bag.
2. If doing anything which will bring you in contact with blood (e.g. surgery or delivering a baby) wear gloves and apron. Protect your eyes with glasses.
3. If blood or other bodily fluid is spilled, clean up as soon as possible. Use an antiseptic, e.g. phenol or sodium hypochlorite.
4. If doing resuscitation **don't** do mouth-to-mouth breathing. Use a bag and mask.

6
Treatment of Tuberculosis

1: GENERAL GUIDE TO TREATMENT

1.1 Introduction

If the doctor prescribes the right medicines, if the patient takes his medicines as prescribed for a sufficiently long period, **all patients should be cured**. The only exception to this rule is if the patient's TB were resistant to the drugs when treatment started.

The **aims of the treatment** are:

1. To cure patients with the least interference with their lives.
2. To prevent death in seriously ill patients.
3. To prevent extensive damage to the lungs with the consequent complications.
4. To avoid relapse of the disease.
5. To prevent the development of resistant tubercle bacilli (acquired resistance).
6. To protect his/her family and the community from infection.

We describe below the drugs which are used in treatment, the regimens (e.g. the drug combinations given; some daily or some several times a week) and the duration of treatment. Before this we will discuss some general points about treatment.

1.2 When to treat (criteria for treatment)

Treatment is expensive. The drugs used can sometimes cause harm to patients. Therefore you should only treat patients who almost certainly have tuberculosis.

Whom should you treat? Clearly patients who are sputum positive on smear examination have top priority. You should also, of course, treat any patient who is found to be positive on culture and any child found to have active disease.

Guidelines for those whom you suspect have tuberculosis but are sputum negative on smear examination are as follows:

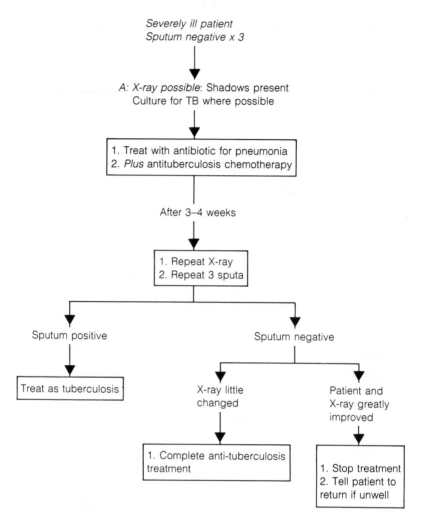

Figure 32a   *Guidelines for managing suspected pulmonary tuberculosis.* **Severely ill patient with 3 sputa negative for TB. X-ray possible** and shows abnormal shadows

If the patient has chest symptoms typical of tuberculosis, but is sputum-negative ×3:

1.2.1   If he is **severely ill** (Figure 32 a and b) and especially if there are abnormal chest signs, get a chest X-ray if possible and start anti-tuberculosis treatment. If pneumonia seems a possibility add a simple antibiotic to treat this.

Examine 3 more sputa for TB. If negative repeat the X-ray in 1 month. If the shadows have mainly cleared, the disease was probably pneu-

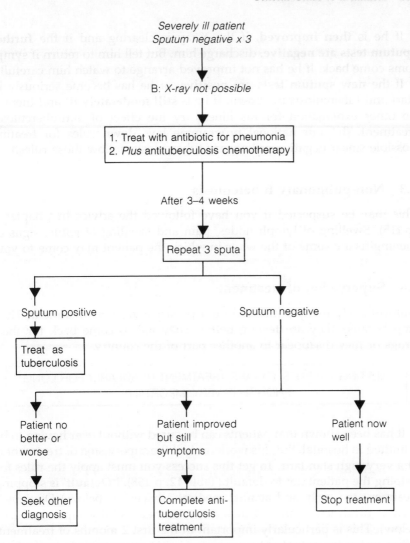

Figure 32b *Guidelines for managing suspected pulmonary tuberculosis.* **Severely ill patient with 3 sputa negative for TB. No X-ray possible**

monia, not tuberculosis. If the patient now seems well, stop treatment. If one of the further sputa proves positive, or tuberculosis still seems probable on clinical grounds, complete treatment.

1.2.2 If he is **not severely ill** (Figure 33, p 157) arrange a chest X-ray if possible. Do a white blood count if possible. Give a trial of non-tuberculous antibiotics (and anti-helminthics in appropriate areas of the world). Review after 3 weeks and repeat sputum ×3 and chest X-ray if possible.

If he is **then improved,** if the X-ray is clearing and if the **further sputum tests are negative,** discharge him. But tell him to return if symptoms come back. If he has not improved arrange to watch him carefully.

If the **new sputum tests are positive,** or he has become seriously ill start anti-tuberculosis treatment. If he is **still moderately ill** and there is no other explanation for his illness try the effect of antituberculosis treatment. (If your national programme lays down rules for treating possible smear-negative pulmonary tuberculosis, follow those rules.)

1.3   Non-pulmonary tuberculosis

This may be suspected if you have followed the advice in Chapter 4 (p 115). Swelling of lymph nodes, pain and swelling of joints, signs of meningitis are some of the ways in which the patient may come to you.

1.4   Supervision of treatment

Unfortunately many patients do not persist with their treatment. They stop because they are feeling better. They fail to come back for their drugs or they disappear to another part of the country.

> GETTING PATIENTS TO TAKE TREATMENT REGULARLY FOR LONG
> ENOUGH IS VERY IMPORTANT.

It has been shown that patients can be cured without ever having to be admitted to hospital. But this works only if the supervision of treatment is of a very high standard. To get this success you must apply the rules for helping the patient not to default (Table 12, p 158). ('**Default**' is stopping treatment too early and against medical advice: see below.) Obviously there is much less chance of default if treatment is fully supervised (see below). This is particularly important in the first 2 months of treatment. Where intensive outpatient supervision is not possible, as in some parts of Africa, much higher rates of cure have been achieved if patients are admitted to a hospital or hostel for the first 8 weeks of treatment. But in many countries this is not possible. See p 159 for other possible forms of supervision.

WHO now recommends for national programmes the 'DOTS' strategy. DOTS stands for 'Directly Observed Treatment Shortcourse'. In this each dose of treatment is supervised by a health professional, other trained worker, or trained volunteer. This is particularly essential in the initial phase of treatment. In those first 2–3 months the most powerful drug combinations are used and most TB are killed. The advantage of this method is that you can be sure that the patient gets every dose. If he fails to come for this dose you can immediately take steps to get him

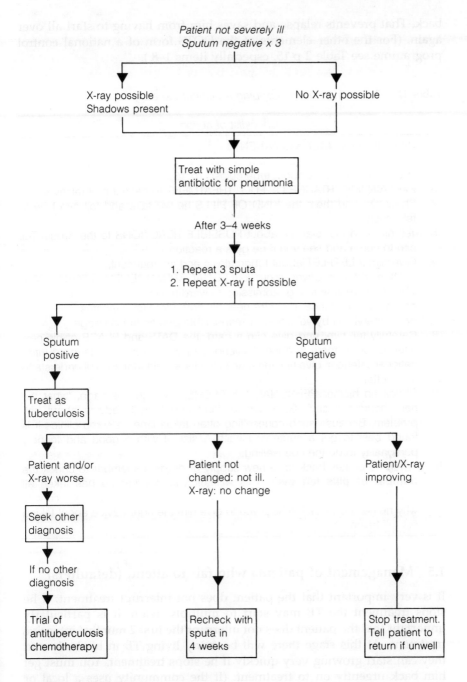

Figure 33 *Guidelines for managing suspected pulmonary tuberculosis.* **Patient not severely ill, 3 sputa negative for TB**

back. That prevents relapse and saves him from having to start all over again. (For the other elements of the DOTS form of a national control programme see Table 2 p 15, especially items 1–8.)

Table 12   *Preventing patient stopping treatment too early*

Checklist of action

1. Be KIND, FRIENDLY and PATIENT.
2. EXPLAIN DISEASE to patient and relatives. In doing this, remember there may be local beliefs about tuberculosis (p 16).
3. EXPLAIN IMPORTANCE OF FULL TREATMENT to patient and relatives.
4. Show him and them the KIND OF PILLS he will take and tell him how to take them.
5. Tell him and his relatives about POSSIBLE REACTIONS to the drugs. Tell him to come and see you if he gets a reaction.
6. Give him a LEAFLET about tuberculosis and its treatment.
7. Tell him and his relatives about your LOCAL ARRANGEMENTS FOR SUPER-VISION of treatment. e.g. admission to ward/hostel
    or   daily attendance at centre near his home for first 2 months
    or   supervision by volunteer or responsible person in his village.
8. Carefully tell him, and give him a card, the DATE and PLACE of his next attendance. If there is a local calendar, different from the standard international calendar, give him the date in the local calendar. He will understand that better.
9. Check on his/her PERSONAL PROBLEMS, e.g. job, marriage, 'what the neighbours will say'. Give him/her kind and friendly advice about any problem. Because such counselling often takes time, in some clinics it is found best to get a nurse or Health Assistant with a good and friendly personality to do the counselling.
10. When he comes back for a new supply of drugs, remember to check the **number of pills left over**. This will tell you whether he has taken all the doses. If he has not taken all the doses, ask him in a sympathetic way why he has not. This will help you to give him the right advice about taking his full treatment.

1.5   Management of patients who fail to attend (defaulters)

It is very important that the patient does not interrupt treatment. If he stops treatment the TB may start to multiply again. It is particularly important that the patient does not interrupt the first 2 months' intensive treatment. At this stage there will be many living TB in his body and they can start growing very quickly if he stops treatment. You must get him back urgently on to treatment. (If the community uses a local or national calendar, remember to give the patient all his appointment dates using that calendar.)

After the first 2 months, in the continuation phase of treatment, it is also important to get him back, but there will be fewer TB and it is less urgent.

We therefore recommend as follows:

1. During the **intensive phase of treatment** when every dose is supervised: if he misses more than one dose take action to get him back.
2. During the **continuation phase of treatment** when the patient is attending monthly: if he fails to attend on the due date take action to get him back.
3. **Action to get patients back**:
   a) It is important to know the patient's correct **address**. For illiterate patients ask him to get his postman to write the address on a card. In order to find the patient easily some clinics ask the patient to give 3 addresses.
   - his home address
   - the address of a friend or relative who lives nearby
   - the address of a shop or restaurant or teahouse which knows the patient and knows where he lives or can be found.

   b) The best and quickest way to get the patient back is by a **home visit** to persuade him to return. This can be done by a specially trained 'home visitor' or 'defaulter tracer'. A good, sympathetic, persuasive personality is important. Alternatively a nurse or other health worker may do it.

   c) **Reminder by post** is less rapid and may be less reliable. It could be the first step for a default in the continuation phase of treatment. If it fails, arrange a home visit. **Default during the intensive phase is dangerous: if at all possible arrange a home visit at once**.

1.6 Preventing the patient stopping treatment too early (preventing default)

There are many aspects of this problem. You must do everything possible to make sure that all your patients take their full treatment. If they do not they are likely to relapse. When you decide to treat a patient, take sufficient time to **talk to him or her** and explain everything in simple terms. Or train a sympathetic nurse or health assistant to do this. If the patient can read **give him a leaflet** which sets out the important details of treatment. (You may be able to get this from your National Tuberculosis Programme or a National Tuberculosis Association.) If he cannot read, someone in his family or village can probably read it to him.

Explain what tuberculosis is and how it can be spread. Reassure him that his disease can be cured if he follows all the advice which you will give him. But tell him that if he does not complete his full treatment the disease is likely to come back.

Show him the **kind of pills** you expect him to take – and show him a second time to make sure he understands. Advise him how often he has to take them. Tell him that even though he begins to feel better he must on no account stop the treatment until the course is finished. In modern treatment there is no need to keep changing drugs: apart from anything else this merely confuses the patient.

Your national programme may have a standard container in which to give the pills to the patient. If possible include 2–3 doses **more** than is needed until he is due to come back for a new supply. This is in case he comes back late. Tell him to **bring back the container** when he returns for his new supply. **Count the remaining pills**. This may tell you whether he has taken all the doses. (Though of course he may have given them away or thrown them away.)

Explain that very rarely patients get a **reaction to drugs** and tell him that the main ones are the return of fever, itching of the skin, rash and, if he is having streptomycin, giddiness. If he is to have ethambutol tell him to report at once if he has difficulty with vision.

One very important reason why a patient may not return to the clinic for his drugs is **economic**. He may not be able to attend during his working hours because he might lose his job and his family could starve. This is particularly important if the clinic is distant, as in rural areas. Try to make arrangements to help the patient avoid this cause of treatment failure.

If possible when the patient returns to the clinic or when he is visited at home, carry out **urine tests** (p 180, 181) for the presence of drugs. At least carry out **pill checks** to see that he has taken the correct number of pills.

Try to get the help of the patient's **relatives and friends**. Explain to them also the way in which the patient should take the drugs. Advise them to keep checking that treatment is being taken regularly and to keep encouraging him throughout treatment.

Advise the patient not to take any medicines for the treatment for tuberculosis which he can buy in the market or be given to him by other 'doctors'. He must not take any additional medicines without consulting you because he might get serious reactions. There is no need to spend money on vitamins, unless they are prescribed by you for a special purpose.

1.7   Where to arrange the treatment centre which the patient will attend for continuation phase of treatment

(The first **intensive** phase must be directly supervised: see p 20 and 156.)

The mistake is sometimes made of arranging this on the outskirts of a town or village. Avoid this, because it will mean patients having to walk long distances.

Choose a clinic which is central, or as near to the patient's home or work as possible. It is useful to have the tuberculosis treatment centre at the same place where people come for other medical purposes, e.g. maternity or immunisation clinics, health posts. For patients in rural areas arrange treatment as near as possible to their home or their work. Time the clinics so that the patient does not have to miss work (see paragraph 1.6 above). Try not to keep patients waiting. If they have long waits they may not come back.

1.8   Choosing staff

If you are able to choose your **staff**, do this with care. Make sure that they treat patients with kindness and understanding. If they are unpleasant the patients may not come back. Choose staff who are keen on their work and who will do the work carefully and with enthusiasm. Encourage them when they do well. If possible one member of staff must undertake clerical duties (keeping of records etc.) and one should act as tracer of missing patients (finding the patients who have failed to return and persuading them to continue treatment).

1.9   Patients' personal problems

Other factors which may interfere with compliance in treatment are **personal problems**, e.g. loss of job and fear about what friends and neighbours will say when they know that the patient has tuberculosis. These are difficult problems but anything that can be done will be helpful in making sure that the patient takes treatment.

1.10   Drug resistance

This is important because treatment will not succeed if the tubercle bacilli are resistant to the drugs used. There are three types of resistance:

1.10.1 Resistant mutants. In any population of TB there will be a small number which are naturally resistant. More of them will occur among the millions of TB in any tuberculous cavity. If only one drug is given the sensitive TB are destroyed but the resistant ones multiply. NEVER GIVE A SINGLE DRUG (MONOTHERAPY).

1.10.2 **Acquired** or **secondary resistance** is caused by

a)   incorrect treatment: e.g. a single drug being given
b)   when two drugs have been given but the patient's bacilli were resistant to one of them, or
c)   the patient failing to take his drugs properly.

1.10.3 **Primary resistance** when the person is infected by someone who has tubercle bacilli with acquired resistance to one or more drugs.

1.11   Follow-up

Sputum tests are more important than X-ray in the follow-up of pulmonary tuberculosis.

Make sure you persuade the patient to come back to the same clinic at regular monthly intervals so that the staff can do urinary tests for the drugs (if this is possible) and check the pills to make sure he is taking everything. This also gives a chance to tell the patient again how important it is to continue treatment even though he is feeling better. And of course he will then be given a new supply of pills.

1.12   Sputum testing

Collect **sputum** from patients for smear examination:

1.   On **short-course chemotherapy** for new patients.
     a)   In 6-month regimen (p 167) test the sputum at the end of the 2nd, 4th and 6th (end of treatment) months.
     b)   In 8-month regimen (p 170) test the sputum at the end of the 2nd, 5th and 8th (end of treatment) months.
2.   If the sputum is **positive at the 2nd month** there are three possibilities:
     a)   Failure to ensure that treatment has been taken as directed. This is far the commonest cause. It may well be a failure to supervise every dose. Look into that very carefully.
     b)   Sometimes it may be due to a slow rate of progress in a patient with extensive disease and a big population of TB.
     c)   Drug resistance is much less likely if you have given one of the standard treatments now recommended (p 167).

If you are sure the patient has taken all his drugs we agree with WHO's recommendation that you give a further month of the full intensive phase treatment.

See p 189 for **how to manage apparent 'failures'**.

Relapse after successful treatment is very rare. You can discharge the patient when the treatment is completed. But tell him to report back if he gets any symptoms.

1.13   Outpatient or hospital treatment

It has been proved conclusively that treatment as an outpatient can be completely successful. The arguments in favour of hospital treatment are that compliance is better, drug toxicity detected earlier, education of patients better, and that isolation means that spread of disease to families and other contacts is less. In fact well-organised clinics can achieve all the benefits which are claimed for hospitalisation. The question of isolation is discussed below.

However, the excellent results have mostly been under ideal conditions where there have been plenty of well-trained staff. Unfortunately in routine service conditions cure rates as low as 30 per cent have been reported. Very rarely have they been higher than 50 per cent. This means not only a poor outcome for individual patients but also means waste of scarce money and resources. **It also means that tuberculosis will not decrease in the community.**

It is calculated that there will only be an important fall in the amount of disease in the community if 85 per cent of patients become sputum negative (75 per cent cure plus an estimated 10 per cent of death). Figures close to this, or even better, have now been achieved by routine services in a number of developing countries. This is especially in the DOTS type of national programme (p 156) started with the help of IUATLD or WHO. The essential is the direct supervision of every dose, at least in the initial intensive phase of treatment. In most programmes this has been outpatient treatment, except for very ill patients. Sometimes, because of distance or other factors, patients have to be admitted to hospital or hostel for the intensive phase. If so, don't assume that if drugs are handed to patients they will be swallowed. Make sure that staff see every dose actually swallowed.

1.14 Isolation

Since good chemotherapy has been started isolation is much less important. There is no increased risk of infection for the family whether the patient is treated at home or in hospital. The greatest risk of infection is before treatment begins. But there are a few groups of patients who may need isolation.

1. **Short-term isolation**: teachers and others in contact with young children.
2. **Isolation until smear negative**: where there is contact with people receiving **immunosuppressive drugs** e.g. anti-cancer drugs; patients who have drug-resistant TB.
3. In hospitals HIV-positive patients who do not have tuberculosis and HIV-positive staff who are still working must be protected from contact with infectious tuberculous patients. Both patients with tuberculosis, and patients admitted for diagnosis who might prove to have tuberculosis, must be in wards where there is no contact with either of these two groups (see p 138).

164 Treatment of Tuberculosis

Infants of tuberculous mothers may die if they are removed from breastfeeding. They should be given preventive treatment with isoniazid (p 165). So should infants in close contact with any sources of infection. You should instruct patients in hospital to **cover their mouths** when coughing. They should cough into disposable tissues. This could be old newspaper which can be burnt. There is no risk of infection from books and personal possessions. If a smear positive patient has been in a room, when he leaves it keep the room unoccupied and well-ventilated for 24 hours. Then clean it thoroughly. For bedding see p 10.

1.15 Contact examination

This is discussed on p 23, paragraph 4.2.11.

1.16 Work

If the patient is not very ill and if he is receiving treatment it has been shown clearly that work is not harmful. It is a great mistake to make the breadwinner stop work because he has tuberculosis. The decision about admission to hospital would partly depend on the severity of the illness, national policy for tuberculosis patients and the economic effects for his family. You must consider all these.

1.17 Lifestyle

It is best to avoid tobacco and alcohol. But it is more important that he should persist with treatment. So don't forbid these if you think it will make him default and fail to take his treatment. After 2–3 weeks the patient is no longer infectious. After that there is no need to alter the degree of sexual activity. However he should avoid any sexual activity which may give a risk of HIV infection (p 136). HIV infection, as well as its bad prognosis, makes permanent cure more difficult. In areas with high HIV incidence counsel the patient how to protect himself/herself by using condoms. Do all that you can do to make condoms available.

1.18 Pregnancy

Pregnancy should probably be avoided during treatment, but there is no need to be anxious if pregnancy does occur. Give pyridoxine (p 180) with isoniazid to avoid any small risk of damaging the infant's nervous system. The other drugs in the routine regimens recommended here are also safe. **But certain drugs should not be given.** Do not give streptomycin (or the reserve drugs capreomycin, kanamycin or viomycin): all these may cause deafness in the infant. Do not give the reserve drugs ethionamide or prothionamide which can cause abnormalities of development in the fetus.

Remember that rifampicin increases the metabolism of oestrogens and this makes contraceptive pill less effective (p 181). Breastfeeding is particularly important when environmental conditions are poor.

1.19   The newborn child

Manage the **newborn child** as follows:

1. **Do not separate the child from the mother** unless she is desperately ill.
2. If the **mother is smear-negative,** give the infant BCG immediately.
3. If the **mother was sputum positive** during pregnancy or is still so at the time of delivery
    a)   if the **infant is ill at birth** and you suspect congenital tuberculosis (p 75) give full anti-tuberculosis treatment
    b)   if the **child is well,** prescribe isoniazid 5 mg/kg in a single dose daily for 2 months. Then do a tuberculin test. If negative stop isoniazid and give BCG. If positive continue isoniazid for a further 4 months. Do not vaccinate with BCG at the same time as isoniazid is being administered. **Or** omit tuberculin test and continue isoniazid for 6 months.
4. In many countries it is safest for the mother to **breast feed** the infant. Breast milk is far the best nutritive for the child. It also protects against many infections. Even if the mother has HIV these advantages are much greater than the small risk of HIV infection by the milk.

2: CHEMOTHERAPY FOR NEWLY DIAGNOSED PATIENTS

2.1   National Tuberculosis Programme

If your country has a National Tuberculosis Programme use the regimen or regimens it recommends. In some programmes the regimens may be different for sputum-negative patients or for children. In some there may be a special retreatment regimen for relapses, defaulters or patients who seem to have failed on the standard regimen for new patients (see p 167, 189). You may find your national regimen or regimens below.

2.2   When there is no National Tuberculosis Programme

If there is no National Programme we recommend that you use one of the regimens included by WHO in its 2nd (1997) edition of *Treatment Guidelines* (p 215 reference 1). The outlines of the different recommended regimens are given in Table 13. You will see that different regimens are recommended according to the type of tuberculosis case.

2.3   Brief method for summarising regimens

The following method is now generally accepted internationally:
   Each standard drug is indicated by a capital letter. They are as follows:

Isoniazid: H	Ethambutol: E
Rifampicin: R	Streptomycin: S
Pyrazinamide: Z	Thioacetazone: T

When the drugs are given daily a figure before the drug combination shows for how many months that combination is given, e.g. 2HRZE indicates that these four drugs are given in a single dose daily for 2 months. Similarly 4HR indicates that these two drugs are given in a single dose daily for 4 months. One of the standard regimens is

2HRZE/4HR

This indicates that the four drugs are given for the first 2 months (known as the **'initial'** or **'intensive phase'**) followed by the two drugs for another 4 months (known as the **'continuation phase'**), making 6 months in all.

In some regimens the drugs are given together in a single dose 3 times a week (**intermittent treatment**). This is indicated by putting the figure 3, lowered by half a space, after each drug. For instance, if the above regimen is given three times weekly instead of daily it is written:

$2H_3R_3Z_3E_3/4H_3R_3$

2.4   Alternative treatment regimens

Alternative treatment regimens recommended by WHO for different treatment categories are shown in Table 13. It is recommended internationally that someone should watch the patient swallow every dose. This is now known as 'DOT', i.e. Directly Observed Treatment. It is especially important in the initial phase. This is to ensure the maximum killing of the millions of TB in the patient at the beginning of treatment (see also p 156).

Table 13   Possible alternative treatment regimens for each treatment category

		Alternative TB treatment regimens	
TB treatment category	TB patients	Initial phase (daily or 3 times per week)	Continuation phase
I	New smear-positive pulmonary TB; new smear-negative pulmonary TB with extensive parenchymal involvement; new cases of severe forms of extrapulmonary TB	2 EHRZ (SHRZ) 2 EHRZ (SHRZ) 2 EHRZ (SHRZ)	6 HE 4HR $4H_3R_3$
II	Sputum smear-positive relapse; treatment failure; treatment after interruption	2 SHRZE/1 HRZE 2 SHRZE/1 HRZE	$5 H_3R_3E_3$ 5 HRE
III	New smear-negative pulmonary TB (other than in Category I); new less severe forms of extra-pulmonary TB	2 HRZ 2 HRZ 2 HRZ	6 HE 4 HR $4 H_3R_3$
IV	Chronic case (still sputum-positive after supervised re-treatment)	NOT APPLICABLE (Refer to WHO guidelines for use of second-line drugs in specialised centres)	

Reproduced with permission of World Health Organization

2.4.1 Intermittent treatment.   You will see in Table 13 that all the regimens can be given either daily or three times a week. But if given three times a week it is particularly essential that **someone watches the patient swallow every dose**. (The supervisor should not be a family member. Experience has shown that family members are much less reliable.) DOT is particularly vital with intermittent treatment. This is because, if a patient misses a dose, the TB will have more time to start to multiply before he comes back for the next dose. Missing doses also risks developing drug resistance. Controlled trials, fully supervised by DOT, have shown that thrice weekly treatment is just as effective as daily treatment. But the dose for most of the drugs must be higher (see Table 14, p 168).

IMPORTANT WARNING ABOUT USING RIFAMPICIN IN THE CONTINUATION PHASE. The IUATLD advises NOT to use rifampicin in the continuation phase UNLESS each dose is DIRECTLY SUPERVISED. Otherwise there is a risk that it may be given in a bad drug combination. Or it may be used for other diseases. Or it may be sold on the black market. All of these risk the development of drug resistance to a very powerful and essential drug. This may easily lead to MULTIPLE DRUG RESISTANCE and so to untreatable disease.

2.4.2 Reason for giving four drugs in the intensive phase. Combined treatment is so effective because for each drug there are a very small number of naturally resistant 'mutant' TB. If the drug is given alone these can survive and multiply to replace the sensitive TB which have been killed by the drug. But the resistant mutants to each drug are killed by the other drugs. Even if the patient has been actually infected by TB resistant to one of the drugs (primary resistance) the other drugs will kill off those resistant bacilli.

2.4.3 We recommend the above regimens for both pulmonary and non-pulmonary tuberculosis in both adults and children. There are some modifications in **tuberculous meningitis: see p 176.**

2.4.4 With any of these regimens if the **sputum is still positive after 2 months, continue the initial four-drug phase for a further month** and then switch to the continuation phase. But **make sure the patient is taking every dose of his treatment.**

2.5   Drug doses

The following dosages (Table 14) have been agreed by international experts. They are approved by WHO and IUATLD.

Table 14   WHO alternative treatment regimens

Drug	Dosage in mg/kg (range)	
	Daily	Thrice/week
Isoniazid	5 (4–6)	10 (8–12)
Rifampicin	10 (8–12)	10 (8–12)
Pyrazinamide	25 (20–30)	35 (30–40)
Streptomycin	15 (12–18)	15 (12–18)
Ethambutol	15 (15–20)	30 (25–35)
Thioacetazone	2.5 (2–3)	Not applicable

Table 15 Fixed-dose drug combinations

Daily treatment

Initial phase

	Drugs		
	R + H + Z	E	S
Dose in 1 tablet (mg)	150 + 75 + 400	400	1 g (vial)
Daily dose (mg)	450 + 225 + 1200	1000	750
No. of tablets	3 tablets	2½ tablets	¾ vial

Continuation phase

	Drugs			
	R + H	E	E + H	Tb1 + H
Dose in 1 tablet (mg)	150 + 75	400	400 + 150	150 + 300
Daily dose (mg)	450 + 225	800	800 + 300	150 + 300
No. of tablets	3 tablets	2 tablets	2 tablets	1 tablet

Intermittent treatment: thrice weekly

Initial phase

	Drugs		
	R + H + Z	E	S
Dose in 1 tablet (mg)	150 + 150 + 500	400	1 g (vial)
Dose (mg)	450 + 450 + 1500	1600	1 g or 750 mg
No. of tablets	3 tablets	4 tablets	1 vial

Continuation phase

	Drugs	
	R + H	E
Dose in 1 tablet (mg)	150 + 150	400
Dose (mg)	450 + 450	1600
No. of tablets	3 tablets	4 tablets

Notes
Rifampicin in patients weighing over 55 kg: add 1 tablet or capsule (150 mg) to the above. This applies both to daily and to intermittent treatment.
Streptomycin dose: for patients over age 60 reduce the dose to 0.5 g (½ vial).

For details about individual drugs see Appendix A p 179.

2.6   Fixed-dose drug combinations (FDCs)

2.6.1   These are now available in many countries. The advantage is that the patient takes all the drugs in the combination together **but** the pills or capsules must be carefully manufactured to make sure that rifampicin is fully absorbed. Each batch should be tested for this. Be careful to use only drugs from a reliable manufacturer.

2.6.2   If you have a National Tuberculosis Control Programme it will give guidance on the number of tablets to be taken. Most patient weigh 45–55 kg. WHO Guidelines gives the examples (listed in Table 15) for this weight.

2.7   8–month regimen avoiding rifampicin in the continuation phase

2.7.1   This involves the use of either thioacetazone (T) or ethambutol in the continuation phase, i.e.

Initial phase: One of the combinations in Table 13 (p 167) followed by for the **continuation phase**:

either	6HT
or	6HE

2.7.2   For the normal adult the dose of T is 150 mg given with 300 mg of H. If E is used, the dose is 800 mg.

2.7.3   The advantage of 6HT is that it is cheap and does not risk wrong use of rifampicin (paragraph 2.4.1 above). The disadvantage is the high risk of dangerous reactions to T if the patient also has HIV infection. As a result some programmes substitute 6HE.

2.7.4   Some countries use the 8–month regimen only for sputum-negative pulmonary tuberculosis or for less ill non-pulmonary disease.

2.8   12-month regimen avoiding rifampicin and pyrazinamide

Some countries still use this regimen. It is cheaper than the short-course regimen, but there are more drug side-effects and usually a higher default rate. Some countries use it only for sputum-negative patients or for less ill non-pulmonary disease. Where HIV is common, it has the important disadvantage of the risk of spreading HIV by streptomycin injections (p 144). There is also the risk of dangerous reactions to thioacetazone (p 184). The regimen is:

2SHT/10HT

2.9 Treatment in special situations

2.9.1 *Pregnant women.* Avoid streptomycin as it may cause deafness in the fetus.

2.9.2. *Women taking the contraceptive pill.* Rifampicin makes the contraceptive pill less effective. It is best if the woman uses another form of contraception while taking rifampicin.

2.9.3 *Patients with liver disorders.* Avoid pyrazinamide. Use one of the following regimens

2SHRE/6HR or 2SHE/10HE

Table 16 Symptom-based approach to adverse effects of TB drugs

Side-effects	Drug(s) probably responsible	Management
Minor		*Continue anti-TB drugs, check drug doses*
Anorexia, nausea, abdominal pain	Rifampicin	Give drugs last thing at night
Joint pains	Pyrazinamide	Aspirin
Burning sensation in the feet	Isoniazid	Pyridoxine 100 mg daily
Orange/red urine	Rifampicin	Reassurance
Major		*Stop responsible drug(s)*
Itching of skin, skin rash	Thioacetazone (streptomycin)	Stop anti-TB drugs (see p 184)
Deafness (no wax on auroscopy)	Steptomycin	Stop streptomycin, use ethambutol
Dizziness (vertigo and nystagmus)	Streptomycin	Stop streptomycin, use ethambutol
Jaundice (other causes excluded)	Most anti-TB drugs (especially isoniazid, pyrazinamide and rifampicin)	Stop anti-TB drugs (see p 188)
Vomiting and confusion (suspect drug induced acute liver failure)	Most anti-TB drugs	Stop anti-TB drugs. Urgent liver function tests and prothrombin time
Visual impairment (other causes excluded)	Ethambutol	Stop ethambutol
Shock, purpura, acute renal failure	Rifampicin	Stop rifampicin

Reproduced with permission of World Health Organization

2.9.4 Patients with renal failure.   Isoniazid, rifampicin and pyrazinamide are either eliminated almost entirely by the bile or get broken down into non-toxic compounds. You can give them in normal dose to patients with renal failure. In severe renal failure, give pyridoxine (p 180) with isoniazid so as to prevent peripheral neuropathy. Streptomycin and ethambutol are excreted by the kidneys. If you can monitor renal function closely it may be possible to give streptomycin and ethambutol in reduced doses. Avoid thioacetazone. It is excreted partially in the urine.

2.10   Watch out for adverse effects of drugs. A symptom-based approach

Adverse effects are shown in Table 16 and are discussed in detail in Reference section pp 179–188.

For management of a patient whose **treatment has apparently failed,** or who has **relapsed,** see p 189.

STORIES ABOUT TREATMENT

Mr Masra

Mr Masra, a **30-year-old man**, had **come up to a health post in a rural area** with cough, sputum and feeling ill for several months. Three sputum specimens were positive for TB. The Health Assistant (HA) put him on **standard treatment** with isoniazid, rifampicin, ethambutol and pyrazinamide. But the HA did not fully explain the treatment to Mr Masra or his family. Mr Masra came back one month later. He was feeling much better and had lost his symptoms. He was given another month's supply of drugs **but then he disappeared**.

Six months later he came back to the health post. He said that 2 months before **his symptoms had come back**. He was **now much more ill**. His **sputum was again positive**. He said that after his last attendance he had felt well and thought he was cured, so he did not come back.

Another HA saw Mr Masra this time. He explained the treatment in a careful and friendly way to both Mr Masra and his wife (p 159). He gave them a leaflet on treatment to take home. Because Mr Masra had previously been taking all the drugs together, while he was still on drugs, the HA knew that the TB should not be resistant. He therefore put him back on the same treatment. He explained that he would have to start from the beginning again and take treatment without any interruption for another full 6 months. At each monthly attendance the HA saw him and talked to him in a friendly careful way. As a result Mr Masra took his treatment equally carefully and was cured.

Comment: The first HA did not take enough trouble to explain all about the treatment to the patient and his family. When the patient failed to come back, the HA did not send anyone to find him. The second HA was quite right in deciding that the patient's TB should be sensitive to all the drugs. He was also quite right to put the patient back on the same treatment. But this time the HA took a lot of trouble to explain everything to the patient and continued to encourage the patient all the way through till he finished his treatment and was cured. Of course it would have been even better if the HA was able to arrange for someone to observe the patient taking every dose of his drugs.

Note: In some national programmes a patient with relapse will be put on one of the standard re-treatment regimens. (See Category II in Table 13, p 167).

Mr Chowdhuri

Mr Chowdhuri, a **man aged forty**, came up to a District Hospital with **cough, sputum and feeling ill**. He said that **2 years before** he was told at a rural health post that he had tuberculosis. He had been given pills for 'several months' and felt better. He then stopped treatment. A few months after this his cough came back and he coughed up some blood. This time he went to a **private doctor** in the nearest town. The doctor gave him some injections. Mr Chowdhuri could only afford the injections for about a month. But his cough disappeared and he felt much better. Now **in the last 2 months all his symptoms had come back**.

The outpatient doctor sent two specimens of **sputum** to be examined for TB. Both were **positive**. The doctor thought that the first treatment had probably been with isoniazid and thioacetazone (Tb1) as that had been the standard health post treatment at the time. The treatment from the private doctor was probably streptomycin injections. He did not seem to have had any other drugs with the injections. (This, of course, was very bad treatment: one drug alone.)

There seemed a possibility that Mr Chowdhuri's TB might be resistant to isoniazid and perhaps to streptomycin. The safest thing was to put him on the standard 5–drug regimen (Table 13 p 167) for re-treatment patients who might have resistant TB. He therefore give him streptomycin, rifampicin, isoniazid and pyrazinamide, with ethambutol as the fifth drug. Streptomycin was given in case his bacilli were still sensitive.

The doctor also took a lot of trouble to explain to Mr Chowdhuri and his wife how important it was to take the 5 drugs with great care for the first 2 months. A Health Assistant watched Mr Chowdhuri swallow the drugs at the time he gave him the streptomycin injection. As he lived close to the hospital he attended for each dose thereafter so as to make sure it was taken as directed. He also told him that if he had any trouble with vision (due to ethambutol: p 183) he should stop treatment and come to see him at once.

The doctor saw Mr Chowdhuri regularly. Each time he talked to him carefully and in a friendly manner. He made sure he knew all about the treatment and how important it was. Mr Chowdhuri soon felt better. He completed treatment and was cured.

3: TREATMENT OF NON-PULMONARY TUBERCULOSIS: MEDICAL TREATMENT

For nearly all these conditions use the same chemotherapy as for pulmonary tuberculosis (p 167). For some of the conditions you should make minor modifications, as follows:

3.1   Pleural effusion

Use standard chemotherapy (p 167). All patients should have full treatment. If not treated 25 per cent of them will later develop tuberculosis in the lungs or elsewhere. If it is available, **prednisolone** (p 188) will make the pleural fluid disappear much more quickly. It will also help to prevent adhesions of the pleural surfaces.

3.2   Pericardial effusion

If you can add prednisolone to the chemotherapy (p 120), it will make it much less likely that the patient will later develop constrictive pericarditis (p 119). It is also much less likely that you will need to repeat needle aspirations of the fluid. Use the standard chemotherapy given on p 167.

3.3   Spinal tuberculosis

Use standard chemotherapy (p 167). Most patients are now treated ambulatory, without bed rest, throughout. But this is unwise if the vertebrae of the neck are involved, because of the severe risk of paralysis of all four limbs. Controlled trials have shown that the disease can always be arrested (stopped) by chemotherapy. But when there is major destruction skilled surgery can reduce later deformity by early **operation**. The surgeon removes abscesses and debris, and follows this by bone grafting. After the operation, the patient has 3–6 weeks rest in bed. Operation may sometimes be needed to release pressure on spinal nerves.
   Tuberculous joints heal well with chemotherapy. Surgical treatment is almost never necessary.

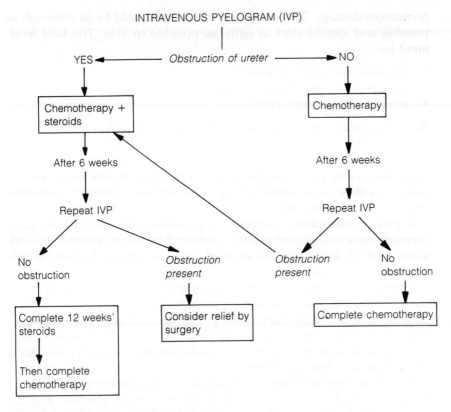

Figure 34 Management of *renal tuberculosis*

3.4 Genito-urinary disease

Use standard chemotherapy. If the ureter becomes obstructed the whole kidney may be lost. Back-pressure from the obstruction may destroy the kidney. To avoid this you have to know what is happening to the ureter. You can only find this out if you have expert radiology and can get intravenous pyelograms. If possible refer the patient to a centre where this can be done. If there is evidence of obstruction, give corticosteroids (as prednisolone) as on p 188). **Figure 34 is a guide to management.**

If it is impossible to get pyelograms, give standard chemotherapy for standard time. You will stop the disease, but the patient may be left with some kidney damage.

3.5 Tuberculous meningitis

Tuberculous meningitis is the most life-threatening of all forms of tuberculosis. It is also the most likely to leave the patient with serious permanent damage. Therefore your treatment should be as thorough as possible and should start as early as possible (p 118). The **best treatment** is:

- isoniazid (10* mg/kg) **with**
- rifampicin (10 mg/kg) **and with**
- pyrazinamide (35 mg/kg).

Add ethambutol (25 mg/kg) **or** streptomycin (10 mg/kg) initially.

For whether to add pyridoxine to isoniazid see p 179.

If the patient makes good progress you can stop streptomycin (or ethambutol) and pyrazinamide after 2–3 months. At this stage you can reduce the dose of isoniazid to 5 mg/kg. Continue rifampicin and isoniazid for at least 9 months.

If you do not have rifampicin or pyrazinamide, give the standard chemotherapy available to you (e.g. isoniazid, streptomycin and thioacetazone: p 170). But make the dose of isoniazid 10 mg/kg for the first 2 months (with pyridoxine if available).

If the patient is making **good progress after 2–3 months,** you can stop the streptomycin. Continue treatment with isoniazid and thioacetazone (at this stage in the standard dose: p 170) for at least a year. It is even better to continue for 18 months to be on the safe side. Many patients do very well with this regimen, though the more intensive treatment above may be somewhat better.

The value of **corticosteroids** (prednisolone) has now been established by a controlled trial. Use it particularly for young children and the severely ill. Begin with 30 mg twice daily (1 mg/kg twice daily for children) for 4 weeks then decrease over several weeks as the patient improves. **For patients on rifampicin the dose should be increased by half,** i.e. 45 mg for adults and 1.5 mg/kg for children. (For the reason see p 189.)

Where you have facilities available **surgery** may be needed to relieve excessive CSF pressure in the ventricles of the brain (hydrocephalus) or to prevent rapid loss of vision. But this should only be done in a special centre.

---

*In India the dose used is 5 mg/kg: the 10 mg/kg dose gives too much toxicity.

REFERENCE SECTION

INTRODUCTION

The rest of this book, Appendices A, B, C, D, E and F, is a REFERENCE SECTION. You can use it to look up particular points when you are faced with a problem. You do not have to remember all the detail. You will find cross-references to this part of the book in various sections of the main text. It is mostly doctors who will use this section. But other health professionals may sometimes wish to look up particular points. Many may find Appendix D on tuberculin testing useful. The Reference Section is arranged as follows:

Appendix A: Some detailed aspects of treatment has four sections.

1. **Drugs used in chemotherapy** (p 179). This gives more detail about each drug.
2. **Management of reactions to antituberculosis drugs** (p 186). Use this section if a patient develops a reaction.
3. **Corticosteroids in the management of tuberculosis** (p 188). This brings together information on use of corticosteroids which is scattered in the various treatment parts of the book.
4. **Management of patients whose chemotherapy has apparently failed** (p 189). Use this if you have to deal with a patient of this kind. It is a common problem.

Appendix B: Surgery in tuberculosis (p 194). This is seldom necessary nowadays. In this part we describe when surgery might sometimes be useful.

Appendix C (p 197): Preventive therapy and chemoprophylaxis. This is not an important part of routine management in high prevalence countries. We outline when it might be used.

Appendix D (p 199): Infections with opportunistic mycobacteria. In countries with a high prevalence of tuberculosis these rarer infections are not important. We describe them briefly. You should refer cases of this kind to an experienced specialist.

Appendix E (p 200) gives more detail about **tuberculin testing**. It includes a description of the technique of the tests and how to read them.

Appendix F (p 206) gives more detail about how to do **gastric suction** in children. For reasons given, this is only used in special cases.

Appendix A
Details of Drug Use

1: DRUGS USED IN CHEMOTHERAPY

This section gives details about the drugs used to treat tuberculosis. Use it for **reference** only.

1.1 General

The drugs commonly available for the treatment of tuberculosis are:

Isoniazid (H)	Pyrazinamide (Z)
Rifampicin (R)	Streptomycin (S)
Ethambutol (E)	Thioacetazone (T)

You will find a summary of side-effects (toxic or adverse effects) of the drugs on p 184, paragraph 1.8.

1.2 Isoniazid

The advantages of isoniazid are that it is a very powerful (bactericidal) drug. It has very few adverse effects. It is very cheap. Because it is so powerful, the dose is small.

It is normally given by mouth. In special circumstances it can be given intravenously and intrathecally. Highly effective concentrations of the drug are obtained in all tissues and the CSF. There is no cross-resistance with other drugs. (The rate of conversion to an inactive form (acetylation) varies in different races but is of no practical importance in standard treatment. However slow inactivators are more likely to get the complication of tingling and numbness of the hands and feet (peripheral neuropathy: see below).)

Preparation and dose.
- Daily: 300 mg (children 5 mg/kg) in a single dose
- Intermittent (× 2/week): 15 mg/kg plus pyridoxine 10 mg with each dose (see below): maximum 750 mg. (× 3/week): 10 mg/kg
- Miliary and meningeal: 5–10 mg/kg (see p 176)
- Chemoprophylaxis: 5 mg/kg
- Intravenously: 200–300 mg (adults) 100–200 mg (children)

The drug is supplied as tablets of isoniazid alone or combined with other drugs (see p 169).

Adverse effects.   Adverse effects of isoniazid are uncommon. Generalised skin rashes rarely occur.

Peripheral neuropathy (tingling and numbness of the hands and feet) is the main adverse effect. It is commoner in malnourished patients and with high doses. It can be treated by giving 100–200 mg pyridoxine daily. It can be prevented by giving 10 mg pyridoxine daily. It is worth giving routine pyridoxine with high dosage isoniazid (for instance in twice weekly treatment): a) if there is much local malnutrition, b) if you are getting many toxic effects and, of course, c) if pyridoxine is available. (Your national programme may make recommendations about this.)

Hepatitis may also occur especially in patients more than 35 years old. Rarer effects are listed on p 185.

Isoniazid **interacts with drugs given for epilepsy** (anti-convulsants) and dosages of these drugs may need to be reduced during chemotherapy.

Test for isoniazid in urine.   The following test is useful where facilities and materials are available. Use a white porcelain plate with small depressions, or something similar. Into each depression put 4 drops of urine, 4 drops of a 10 per cent solution of potassium cyanide (Caution: Poison) and then 10 drops of 10 per cent chloramine T without shaking the plate. A pink or red colour indicates that isoniazid is present. The test is positive for at least 12 hours after a dose. The reagents used should be prepared weekly and kept in a refrigerator.

1.3   Rifampicin

Rifampicin is always given by the mouth in a single dose. There is no cross-resistance to other anti-tuberculosis drugs. Highly effective concentrations are obtained in all tissues and moderate levels in the CSF. Although the cost is higher than most other usual drugs, the results are so good that chemotherapy may be cheaper per cured case (see p 170).

Preparation and dose.
* Daily: 55 kg body-weight and over: 600 mg
  under 55 kg: 450 mg
  (10 mg/kg, maximum)
  children   10 mg/kg
  (maximum   450 mg)
* Intermittent (p 169): 450 mg twice or thrice weekly

It should, if possible, be taken half an hour before breakfast. If nausea is a problem, it should be taken last thing at night.

It is supplied as capsules or tablets, (syrup is also available) either alone or combined with other drugs (see p 169).

An intravenous preparation is available.

You should warn all patients that **rifampicin colours the urine, sweat and tears pink**.

Adverse reactions.   The main side-effects when the drug is given daily are **gastro-intestinal**: nausea, anorexia and mild abdominal pain, diarrhoea occurring less frequently. You can often get over these problems by giving it last thing at night.

Cutaneous reactions in the form of mild flushing and itchiness of the skin, and occasionally a rash, occur very infrequently. These reactions are often so mild that the patient desensitises himself without the drug having to be stopped.

Hepatitis is extremely uncommon unless the patient has a history of liver disease or alcoholism. It is wise if possible to estimate liver function from time to time in such patients. A significant rise in bilirubin may occur in patients with congestive cardiac failure.

The following patterns of adverse effects (syndromes) occur mostly in patients having **intermittent treatment**. They may also rarely occur in patients who have been **prescribed** daily treatment but **take** the drugs intermittently.

1. 'Influenza' syndrome, shiveriness, malaise, headache and bone pain.
2. Thrombocytopenia and purpura: platelets fall to a very low level and haemorrhages occur. It is essential to stop treatment immediately.
3. Respiratory and shock syndrome: shortness of breath, wheeziness, fall in blood pressure, collapse. Corticosteroids may be required.
4. Acute haemolytic anaemia and renal failure.

Rifampicin should never be given again if the shock syndrome, acute haemolytic anaemia or acute renal failure has occurred.

Rifampicin and other drugs.   Rifampicin stimulates liver enzymes which may break down other drugs more rapidly than normal. This includes the oestrogens in the contraceptive pill. You must advise other forms of contraception in female patients receiving rifampicin. You may have to give higher doses of certain drugs if the patient is also receiving rifampicin. But remember to reduce the dose when the patient ceases to take rifampicin. These drugs include oral coumarin anticoagulants, oral diabetic drugs, digoxin, methadone, morphine, phenobarbitone and dapsone.

Test for rifampicin in the urine.   Rifampicin can be identified in the urine by a simple test. Mix 10 ml of urine with 2 ml chloroform (analytical grade) by tilting gently in a screw-topped tube. The test is negative if no colour develops: a yellow to orange colour developing in the chloroform layer indicates the presence of rifampicin. The test will detect rifampicin for 6 hours, and in some patients up to 12 hours, after taking rifampicin. Tetracyclines also give a yellow colour. A cruder test is just to look for the red colour in the urine.

1.4   Streptomycin

Streptomycin is not absorbed from the intestine so you have to give it by intramuscular injection. It diffuses readily into most body tissues. The concentrations are very low in normal CSF (cerebrospinal fluid) but the levels are higher if there is meningitis. It does however cross the placenta. As it is excreted almost entirely through the kidney the dosage has to be lowered in patients with poor renal function and in older age groups. Providing syringes and staff to inject the drug add to the cost.

Preparation and dosage.   Streptomycin sulphate for intramuscular injection is supplied as a powder in vials. It is made into a solution by adding distilled water. Ideally, solutions should be prepared immediately before administration.

Make sure the nurse gives the injection into a different site each day. Daily injections into the same site are very **painful**. Because it is painful, only give streptomycin to **children** if it is essential.

The **nurse** who gives the injections must wear gloves. Otherwise there is a risk of her developing **skin reactions** to the streptomycin.

HIV can be spread by infected needles. If you cannot use a new needle for every patient, or if you cannot be sure that sterilisation is absolutely reliable, you should substitute ethambutol for streptomycin. This is particularly important if you are working in an area which has a high prevalence of AIDS. (But do not use ethambutol in young children: they may not tell you if they are losing vision.)

Dosage

Adults (daily)	below age of 40 years	
	weight under 50 kg:	0.75 g in a single dose
	over 50 kg:	1.0 g
	between 40–60 years	0.75 g
	over 60 years	0.5 g
Children (daily)		10 mg/kg not exceeding 0.75 g
Intermittent:	less than 50 kg	0.75 g
	50 kg or more	1.0 g
	children	15 mg/kg: not exceeding 0.75 g

Adverse effects.   The main adverse effects are cutaneous hypersensitivity and ototoxicity (damage to eighth nerve).

Skin reactions – rash and fever – usually occur in the second and third weeks. Their management is described on p 186.

Damage to the vestibular (balancing) apparatus is shown by giddiness. It may start suddenly and, if acute, there may also be vomiting. Unsteadiness is more marked in darkness. Examination of the eyes may show nystagmus. It is more likely to occur in older patients: attention to dosage is very important. **Treatment must be stopped immediately**. The damage to the nerve may be permanent if the drug is not stopped when the symptoms start. If the drug is stopped immediately symptoms usually clear over weeks. **Deafness** occurs extremely rarely.

Anaphylaxis: injection may be followed by tingling around the mouth, nausea and occasionally by sudden collapse. Streptomycin **should be avoided**, if at all possible, in **pregnancy** because it may cause **deafness** in the child.

1.5 Ethambutol

Ethambutol is a bacteriostatic drug. It is mainly used to prevent the emergence of drug resistance to the main bactericidal drugs (isoniazid, rifampicin and streptomycin). It is given orally.

Preparation and dosage. Because of the risk of blindness large doses are no longer given. **You must make sure not to give more than the recommended dose.** Never give ethambutol to young children who are unlikely to tell you they are losing their sight.

Dosage

Adults (daily):	25 mg/kg **for the first 8 weeks only**
	15 mg/kg subsequently
Adults (3 × week)	30 mg/kg
(2 × week)	45 mg/kg

Avoid in young children and renal failure.

Adverse reactions. The main and possibly very serious, adverse reaction is **progressive loss of vision** caused by retrobulbar neuritis. When you start the patient on treatment **warn him about possible decrease in vision.** The patient will notice failing eyesight even before anything shows in the eye when you examine it with the ophthalmoscope. He must stop the drug immediately. If he does this there is every chance that he will recover his sight. If he continues the treatment he may become completely blind. Eye damage is much more common if the patient has renal failure. For rarer adverse effects see p 185.

1.6 Pyrazinamide

Pyrazinamide is a highly bactericidal drug. It is particularly effective in killing off TB inside cells. It is very valuable in short-course treatment and in meningitis.

Treatment and dosage. It is administered by mouth: each tablet contains 400 or 500 mg pyrazinamide: it should be taken in a single dose.

Adults (daily)	25 mg/kg (20–30 mg)
(3 × weekly)	35 mg/kg (30–40 mg)
(2 × weekly)	50 mg/kg (40–60 mg)
Children (daily)	
(3 × weekly)	} As above
(2 × weekly)	

Adverse effects. The commonest side-effects are liver damage (hepatotoxicity) and pain in the joints (arthralgia). **Hepatotoxicity** may be discovered only on carrying out routine biochemical tests. Anorexia, mild fever, tender enlargement of liver and spleen may be followed by jaundice. If severe hepatitis occurs do not give the drug again.

Arthralgia is quite common and is often mild. The pain affects both large and small joints – shoulders, knees and fingers especially. The level of uric acid is increased and gout may occur. Simple treatment with aspirin is often sufficient: allopurinol is required for the treatment of gout. Rarer side effects are listed on p 185.

1.7   Thioacetazone (Tb1)

Thioacetazone is a weak drug but is very valuable as a companion drug in preventing the development of isoniazid resistance. It is relatively cheap and remains stable in high temperatures. It is poorly tolerated by the Chinese population of Hong Kong and Singapore, poorly tolerated by Europeans and surprisingly well tolerated in East African countries and in South America. (But severe reactions may occur in patients with HIV infection.) Natural resistance to thioacetazone occurs in certain countries. It should be used only in communities where it has been shown to be effective and to be of low toxicity.

Preparation and dosage.   You must give thioacetazone in a single dose daily. Make sure you give exactly the right dose. Too small a dose will fail to prevent resistance. It is unsuitable for intermittent use. Combined preparations with isoniazid are available. Avoid using the drug in liver disease and renal failure.

Dosage

Adults (daily)	150 mg
Children (daily)	2.5 mg/kg (max 150 mg)
Intermittent	unsuitable

Adverse effects.   The main adverse effects are generalised cutaneous reactions and gastro-intestinal symptoms. These are very common in patients with HIV infection and may be very severe. For management see p 186.

Fever and **rash** are sometimes severe and exfoliation of skin may occur.

Gastro-intestinal symptoms include nausea, abdominal discomfort and vomiting.

Rarer side-effects are listed on p 185.

1.8   Summary of toxic reactions to the main anti-tuberculosis drugs

Rifampicin

Uncommon: hepatitis, cutaneous reactions, gastrointestinal reactions, thrombocytopenic purpura; febrile reactions ('influenza' syndrome) during intermittent or irregular administration.

Rare (usually during intermittent or irregular administration): shortness of breath, shock, haemolytic anaemia, acute renal failure.

Toxic reactions are rare in children.

Isoniazid
Uncommon: hepatitis, cutaneous hypersensitivity, peripheral neuropathy (preventable and treatable with pyridoxine).
Rare: giddiness, convulsions, optic neuritis, mental symptoms, haemolytic anaemia, aplastic anaemia, agranulocytosis, lupoid reactions, arthralgia, gynaecomastia.

Ethambutol
Uncommon: retrobulbar neuritis (dose-related), arthralgia
Rare: hepatitis, cutaneous hypersensitivity, peripheral neuropathy.

Pyrazinamide
Common: anorexia, nausea, flushing.
Uncommon: hepatitis (dose-related), vomiting, arthralgia, skin rashes (especially when exposed to sun).

Streptomycin
Common: Cutaneous hypersensitivity, giddiness, numbness, tinnitus.
Uncommon: vertigo, ataxia, deafness.

Thioacetazone
Common: gastro-intestinal reactions, cutaneous hypersensitivity, vertigo, conjunctivitis.
Uncommon: hepatitis, erythema multiforme, exfoliative dermatitis (more common in some populations than in others), haemolytic anaemia.
Rare: agranulocytosis.

1.9 'Second-line drugs'

These drugs are used for patients whose bacilli have been proved to be resistant to all the five standard drugs. They are very difficult to use. They have many side-effects. They are less effective and very expensive. An experienced specialist has to work out the best drug combinations for each patient. WHO recommends that the drugs should only be used in specialist centres. For guidance for these centres see Crofton J., Chaulet P., Maher D. *Guidelines for the Management of Drug-resistant Tuberculosis*. Geneva: WHO, 1997. See also p 189 and 192.

The following drugs have been used for this purpose. The names are only given here for reference.

Ethionamide
Prothionamide
Sodium para-aminosalicylate (PAS)
Cycloserine
Ofloxacin

Capreomycin
Kanamycin
Viomycin
Amikacin
Ciprofloxacin

2: MANAGEMENT OF REACTIONS TO ANTI-TUBERCULOSIS DRUGS

These are important because they cause discomfort to patients and because they interrupt treatment.

2.1   Hypersensitivity (allergic) reactions

These rarely occur in the first week of treatment. They are commonest in the second to fourth week. They are much less frequent with isoniazid, rifampicin and ethambutol than they are with streptomycin and thioacetazone. Very rarely patients become allergic to all three drugs in a regimen.

There are various degrees of reaction:

1. **Mild**: itching of the skin only: this is often the only sign of rifampicin allergy.
2. **Moderate**: fever and rash. The rash is often mistaken for measles or scarlet fever. If severe the skin looks blistered and resembles urticaria.
3. **Severe**: In addition to fever and rash there may be generalised swelling of lymph nodes, enlargement of liver and spleen, swelling round the eyes and swelling of the mucous membranes of the mouth and lips. High fever, a generalised blistering rash and ulceration of the mucous membranes of the mouth, genitals and eyes (Stevens–Johnson syndrome). This is a rare but dangerous reaction, particularly to thioacetazone, and particularly in patients with HIV infection. Very rarely there may be chronic eczema involving the limbs occurring after the eighth week. This is almost always due to allergy to streptomycin.

Management.   This is discussed in two parts: immediate and desensitisation.

Immediate.   If the only complaint is **mild itching** you can usually continue drug treatment, as the patient desensitises himself; give anti-histamine drug (if available). **But if patient receiving Tb1** and might be HIV positive, **stop Tb1 at once.** Never give it again. Substitute ethambutol.

If there is **fever** and **rash**, stop all drugs; give anti-histamine drug (if available). If there is a **very severe reaction**, stop all drugs.

If the patient seems seriously ill, it may be necessary to send the patient to hospital for treatment with:

* hydrocortisone 200 mg IV or IM, then
* dexamethasone 4 mg IV or IM until the patient can swallow, then
* prednisolone 15 mg three times a day orally, reducing the dose gradually every two days depending upon the patient's response
* IV fluids if required.

Desensitisation should NOT be tried if the patient has had a very severe reaction.

Desensitisation.   This should not be begun until the hypersensitivity reaction has disappeared. Management of desensitisation is best done in hospital.

If possible give two anti-tuberculosis drugs which the patient has not pre-viously received while you are carrying out desensitisation.

Start giving test doses as shown in Table 17. Thioacetazone and streptomycin are the most likely to produce an allergic reaction: test for them last. The reaction is usually a slight skin rash or slight fever. It usually shows within 2–3 hours. You can therefore test two doses a day, at 12-hour intervals, if the patient is in a hospital or a hostel.

With the increase of HIV and the risk of dangerous reactions from thioaceta-zone **don't attempt to desensitise** to that drug. If HIV is a risk in your area **don't even give a test dose of thioacetazone**. Substitute ethambutol. Test all drugs the patient has received before starting desensitisation because you may be able to give two of the drugs while desensitising to the third.

There are so many effective drugs now that, if you have other drugs available, it is often easier to substitute another drug for the one which has caused the reaction. **Check that if you do substitute a drug that this does not mean that you need to change from a short-course (6 month) regimen to treatment for 12 months**. If you do not have alternative drugs, below is a guide to desensitisa-tion.

Table 17 *Challenge doses for detecting cutaneous or generalised hypersensiti-vity to anti-tuberculosis drugs*

Drug	Challenge doses	
	Day 1	Day 2
Isoniazid	50 mg	300 mg
Rifampicin	75 mg	300 mg
Pyrazinamide	250 mg	1.0 g
Ethambutol	100 mg	500 mg
Thioacetazone	25 mg	50 mg
Streptomycin or other aminoglycosides	125 mg	500 mg

Reproduced with permission from Girling, D. J. Adverse effects of anti-tuberculosis drugs. *Drugs*, 1982; **23**: 56–74.

If a reaction occurs with the **first challenge dose** drug (as shown on Table 17) you know the patient is hypersensitive to that drug. When starting to desensitise it is usually safe to **begin with a tenth of the normal dose**. Then increase the dose by a tenth each day. If he has a mild reaction to a dose, give the same dose (instead of a higher dose) next day. If there is no reaction, go on increasing by a tenth each day. If the reaction is severe (which is unusual) go back to a lower dose and increase the doses more gradually.

If the patient is in hospital, or can attend at 12 hourly intervals, you can give the doses twice a day and save time. In most cases you can easily complete the desensitisation within 7–10 days.

As soon as you have completed the desensitisation to that drug, begin giving it regularly but make sure that it is combined with at least one other drug (to which the patient is **not** hypersensitive) so as to prevent drug resistance.

2.2 Hepatitis

All anti-tuberculosis drugs can cause damage to the liver, ethambutol and cyclo-serine very rarely. It is very difficult to decide whether hepatitis is due to drugs or to infectious hepatitis in countries where this disease may be common. Hepatitis as a side-effect probably occurs in about 1 per cent of treated patients, and is probably commonest with thioacetazone and pyrazinamide.

Mild symptomless increase in serum enzymes is a common occurrence. This is not an indication to stop drugs. If there is loss of appetite, jaundice and liver enlargement, treatment should be stopped until liver function has returned to normal. Strangely enough in most patients the same drugs can be given again without return of hepatitis.

If the hepatitis has been severe don't use pyrazinamide or rifampicin for retreatment. Give streptomycin, isoniazid and ethambutol for 2 months, followed by **10 months** of isoniazid and ethambutol (2SHE/10HE).

If the patient is severely ill with tuberculosis and might die without chemo-therapy, it is safest to give streptomycin and ethambutol (the least hepatotoxic drugs). When the hepatitis has settled restart standard chemotherapy unless the hepatitis has been very severe. If hepatitis has been severe, use 2SHE/10HE as above.

3: CORTICOSTEROIDS IN THE MANAGEMENT OF TUBERCULOSIS

Corticosteroids suppress the inflammatory response to injury or infection. They can therefore not only help in treatment but may also be harmful. NEVER GIVE CORTICOSTEROIDS in tuberculosis or suspected tuberculosis UNLESS THE PATIENT IS ALSO TAKING EFFECTIVE ANTI-TUBERCULOSIS DRUGS. The only possible exception is the treatment of a severe allergic reaction to drugs (p 186).

3.1 Possible indications for corticosteroid drugs in tuberculosis

1. They are definitely useful in the treatment of severe **allergic reactions** (hypersensitivity) to drugs (p 186), including patients with HIV infection and tuberculosis.
2. They are useful in reducing the out-pouring of fluid from serous surfaces – **pleural effusion** (p 174), **pericardial effusion** with much fluid (p 174) and **peritoneal effusion** (p 129).
3. They help to reduce **fibrosis** and scar tissue e.g. in tuberculosis of the **eye** (p 69), the **larynx** (p 115) and obstruction of the ureter in **renal** tuberculosis (p 175).
4. Their value in **tuberculous meningitis** has now been proved (p 176).
5. Do not give corticosteroids routinely to patients with **pulmonary tubercu-losis**. But if you have these drugs and the patient seems so ill that he might

die within the first few days of chemotherapy, then corticosteroids may keep him alive until the drugs begin to work.

6. In disease of the **adrenals** (Addison's disease), you have to replace the missing adrenocorticotrophic hormones (p 130).

If you are not very experienced and do not know whether you should give corticosteroids or not, and if a senior colleague is available, ASK ADVICE. Only give these drugs under medical supervision and in hospital.

3.2 Precautions

Remember that corticosteroids cause ill-effects such as fluid retention, moon-face, mental symptoms occasionally and worsening of a gastric or duodenal ulcer. In tuberculosis corticosteroids (such as prednisolone) only have to be given for some weeks or at most a month or two. Therefore, long-term ill-effects (high blood pressure, diabetes, softening of the bones) should not occur.

3.3 Dosage

In mild conditions an initial dose of prednisolone 10 mg twice daily for 4–6 weeks is usually enough. After that reduce the daily dose by 5 mg each week.

In seriously ill patients the dose should be as follows:

- **Tuberculous meningitis** 30 mg twice daily for 4 weeks, then decrease gradually over several weeks according to progress.
- **Tuberculous pericarditis** 30 mg twice daily for 4 weeks, 15 mg twice daily for the second 4 weeks and then decrease gradually over several weeks.
- **Tuberculous pleural effusion** 20 mg twice daily for 2 weeks, and then decreasing rapidly. The dose for children is 1–3 mg/kg daily, divided into two equal doses. The higher dose would be for the more severely ill child.
- **In patients receiving rifampicin the dose should be increased by half for the first 2–4 weeks**. The reason is that RIF antagonises the action of prednisolone.

Steroids suppress the immune processes. So of course does HIV. But on balance patients with the above conditions are likely to benefit from the use of steroids so do use if for these patients.

4: MANAGEMENT OF PATIENTS WHOSE CHEMOTHERAPY HAS APPARENTLY FAILED

4.1 Suspecting treatment failure

There are two situations in which you might suspect treatment failure:

1. The patient is supposed to be taking treatment but sputum smears remain positive at 5–6 months. Or the patient's smear was negative at, perhaps, the second and third month but is again positive at 5–6 months ('fall and rise phenomenon').

2. The patient is supposed to have completed treatment but comes back to a clinic and is found to be sputum smear positive again (apparent relapse).

4.2 Investigations

When either 1. or 2. above has happened, do not alter treatment without making certain investigations:

1. Find out **what treatment he has had** – the drugs, the doses, the rhythm, the duration and whether it was supervised or not. If possible get the information from his clinic record card: for instance this may show that he defaulted at a certain time or that pill collection was irregular. It is a good idea to write the information down on a piece of paper: it often helps you to see the problem more clearly!
2. If the reason for failure is not obvious from the records, explain to the patient that he is positive (either remains positive or has again become positive). Speak to him kindly and say that to give him the best treatment now you must know what has happened: has he taken **all his pills all the time**? If not, did he miss taking them for days, weeks or months at a time? If he claims he did take all the pills all the time, try to **interview a reliable member of his family** (without the patient being there). A relative is often more truthful, as naturally patients do not want it known that what has gone wrong could be their own fault (though **your** proper attitude is that it is your fault for not fully motivating the patient and his family!). Again, write down the result of your enquiries.
3. Consider the possibility of **HIV infection**. Although most HIV infected patients with tuberculosis do respond to treatment, they can relapse. Take a careful history and examine the patient for other signs of HIV infection. Counsel the patient and test for HIV antibodies if this test is available and if the patient agrees (p 142).
4. If you have a reliable reference laboratory you can send sputum specimens for culture and sensitivity patterns. In most places this will not be possible. In any case it will take weeks to get the results and you need to make a decision soon about treatment in most cases.

4.3 Too short treatment

If the patient has stopped treatment after too short a period, and has been given one of the recommended regimens, he will be **relapsing with sensitive TB**. The same is true if he has had one of the recommended short course regimens and has apparently responded well to treatment, but is now sputum positive again. In either case you can treat him again with the same combination of drugs. But if there is any question that he took his drugs irregularly, or took some drugs but not others, his bacilli may be resistant to one or more of the drugs. As it may be difficult to be sure of what he has taken, WHO now recommends that all relapsing patients be put on one of the standard retreatment regimens (Table 13, Treatment Category II, p 167 or 4.5 below). If he has relapsed after apparently taking the full standard course of therapy, also put him on one of the standard retreatment regimens. In practice most such patients do not have drug resistance.

Relapse is due to incomplete treatment, but the patient had failed to tell you this.

4.4   Probable drug resistance

If a patient fails to improve and remains sputum positive for 5–6 months, but you are quite sure he is taking all his drugs regularly, this means that his TB have probably been resistant right from the start of treatment. If his sputum first becomes negative but later becomes positive again (and you are quite sure he is taking all his drugs) this means that his TB were resistant to one or more of the drugs to begin with and have now become resistant to the other drugs you are using. If either of these happens it is necessary to change the treatment.

4.5   Managing the patient with relapse

As mentioned in 4.3 above, WHO now recommends two alternative regimens which should cure most patients with relapse, whether due to too short treatment or to drug resistance. (See Category II in Table 13, p 167 and 4.5.2 below.)

The treatment WHO recommends may only fail in patients who have had repeated courses of several drugs, either alone or in bad combinations.

In these relapsed patients you must make sure the patient takes every dose, especially in the first 2–3 months. **This may be his last chance of cure.** So the patient must either be admitted to a hospital or hostel, or must attend a clinic or Health Post for every dose.

4.5.1 Definition of relapse.   A patient who **now has positive sputum smears** AND **either** has **completed** a full course of chemotherapy **and** become direct smear and/or culture negative **or** has had sufficient chemotherapy to become direct smear and/or culture negative.

4.5.2 Recommended retreatment regimens.   WHO recommends these for sputum positive patients who have either (a) relapsed or (b) failed to respond to a standard regimen recommended for new patients (i.e. still remaining sputum positive at the end of a supposed standard course). In practice many of the apparent failures turn out not to have drug resistance. Treatment in fact has been incomplete.

The regimens are:

either streptomycin plus isoniazid plus rifampicin plus pyrazinamide plus ethambutol, given daily in a single dose for 2 months
  * streptomycin is then stopped and the other 4 drugs continued in a single daily dose for a further 1 month
  * pyrazinamide is then stopped and the other 3 drugs continued in a single daily dose for a further 5 months, making 8 months in all

or the same regimen for the first 3 months, followed by
  * isoniazid, rifampicin, and ethambutol in a single dose 3 times a week for the last 5 months.

These regimens may be summarised (as in Table 13 p 167) as

2SHRZE/1HRZE/5HRE

or

2SHRZE/1HRZE/5H$_3$R$_3$E$_3$

Both of these regimens may be given in a single dose 3 times a week throughout the full 8 months (with the correct change in dosage for intermittent treatment: see p 168 and following pages).

This is the patient's last chance of cure. **You must make sure that he is seen to swallow every dose.** This may mean that the patient has to be in hospital or hostel throughout.

4.5.3 *Monitoring treatment.* Examine the sputum for positivity at the end of the 3rd, 5th, and 8th months (end of treatment).

- **If still positive at 3 months.** Continue the 4 drugs for another month and then start the continuation phase. Make sure he is taking every dose.
- Retest at 4 months: if still positive get culture and sensitivity tests done if possible. But go ahead with the continuation phase.
- If shown to have resistance to 2 or more of the drugs used in the continuation phase: refer to a special centre for multiresistant patients (see 4.6 below). If no special centre, continue to end of retreatment regimen: make sure he takes every dose.
- If still positive at 8 months (end of treatment): refer to special centre if available.

4.5.4 *Results.* One of the above regimens should cure most patients with relapse. It should also cure most patients after apparent failure of a standard regimen for new patients (p 167). It may cure some of the patients with a history of repeated, and probably unreliable, treatment: the 'chronic' patients. It may fail in some of these patients, if there is already resistance to most of the drugs used: Multidrug Resistance (MDR). Therefore you should refer such 'chronic patients' to a special centre if available (see 4.6 below). If there is no special centre, the best you can do is to give one of the standard retreatment regimens in 4.5.2 above.

4.6   Probable multiple drug resistance

1. Unfortunately this is a problem which may be common in some countries. It is usually due to private doctors giving short courses of a single drug (often rifampicin) or drugs in bad combinations. The doctor may have given, or added, a new drug each time the patient has relapsed.
2. If there is resistance to 1 or 2 standard drugs the treatment given in paragraph 4.5 should cure the patient.
3. If previous treatment suggests resistance to isoniazid, rifampicin and streptomycin, **treatment is very difficult.** The reserve drugs (p 185) are weaker and have many side-effects. **If possible refer the patient to a specialist centre.**
4. The specialist will start with 4 or 5 drugs. He will use drugs the patient has

not had before, or drugs already used but to which the patient's bacilli are probably sensitive. When the sputum has become negative he will stop 1 or 2 of the weaker or toxic drugs. He will continue treatment for at least 18 months. This treatment can be successful, but it needs very skilful supervision and encouragement of the patient to tolerate the unpleasant side-effects of the drugs.

5. In some countries it is now difficult to obtain certain of these reserve drugs. The specialist will have to use what is available.

6. As such treatment is expensive, highly specialised and very difficult, some national control programmes have to regard these patients as untreatable. Resources should concentrate on giving good standard treatment to all new patients. Good standard treatment does not give rise to drug resistance. However some richer countries may be able to afford enough finance and highly specialised training to provide a specialist centre (perhaps more than one in big countries) where such patients may be treated. WHO has now produced special guidelines, but these are designed only for such specialist centres: See *Guidelines for the Management of Drug-resistant Tuberculosis*: Reference 5, p 215.

Appendix B
Surgery in Tuberculosis

Chemotherapy is now so effective that surgery is rarely needed. In well-equipped and well-staffed centres it might occasionally be useful, as listed below. **But you should be able to cure almost all your tuberculosis patients without it.**

1: PLEURO-PULMONARY DISEASE

1. Very **unco-operative patients** who continue to spread their infection in the community.
2. Resection of lung in patients with **drug-resistant TB** who have failed on re-treatment with reserve drugs. (Most of these patients will have too extensive lung destruction to be suitable for surgery. In any case surgery is highly dangerous unless there are at least two reserve drugs to cover the operation and the postoperative period.)
3. Patients whose tuberculosis had been cured but nevertheless have recurrent **severe haemoptysis** from an open cavity or bronchiectasis. This may follow infection of an open cavity with the fungus *Aspergillus fumigatus* (p 103).
4. Very rarely, in children and young adults, surgical removal of mediastinal glands pressing on trachea and large bronchi is required – sometimes as an emergency.
5. Surgical removal of a tuberculous empyema (p 106) which has failed to clear.
6. If there is a round solid (coin) lesion in the lung there is sometimes doubt as to whether it is a tuberculoma or a tumour. It is best to remove it.

2: LYMPH NODE DISEASE (pp 56, 122)

Surgical removal of lymph nodes is very seldom needed nowadays. Occasionally it is useful for diagnosis if the cause of the lymph node enlargement in a patient is very difficult to decide. Of course it is only useful to remove the lymph node if you have facilities for histological examination. If you cannot do histology and you strongly suspect tuberculosis, try the effect of anti-tuberculosis chemotherapy. There is no place now for the block removal of groups of nodes in the neck. It is better to incise a lymph node abscess and remove its contents rather than to aspirate it by needle.

3: BONE AND JOINT DISEASE (p 62)

1. **Spinal tuberculosis**. Surgical treatment is seldom essential. It is occasionally needed when collapse of vertebrae and collections of caseous material produce or threaten paralysis of limbs. If these are not relieved with treatment within a week to ten days, consider surgery if this is available. But remember surgery can reduce later deformity (see p 174).
2. **Tuberculosis of joints** (p 174) responds very well to chemotherapy; surgery is required only exceptionally.

4: GENITO-URINARY DISEASE

1. If **renal tuberculosis** (p 175) is managed properly with chemotherapy and, where appropriate, **corticosteroids**, removal of a kidney should hardly ever be necessary.
2. Resection of **testis** or **epididymis** (p 128) should never be carried out unless there is doubt about the diagnosis, and you suspect a possible cancer.
3. Reconstruction of the **fallopian tube** (p 127) is an operation for a very specialised surgeon.

5: ABDOMINAL TUBERCULOSIS (p 129)

This form of the disease responds very well to chemotherapy. The abdominal contents are usually so matted together that any operation is very difficult and risky. An operation is sometimes necessary to relieve intestinal obstruction caused by residual adhesions.

6: TUBERCULOSIS OF THE THYROID AND BREAST

Surgical removal of a mass may be carried out because the diagnosis is in doubt, and you suspect a possible cancer.

7: TUBERCULOSIS OF THE PERICARDIUM (p 120)

1. Open drainage is seldom necessary in the acute stage.
2. Removal of a thickened and partly calcified pericardium may be needed if, in the process of healing, the disease causes constriction of the heart, and interferes with its proper action (p 120).

Appendix C
Preventive Therapy and Chemoprophylaxis

For some time most experts thought that there was no place for preventive therapy and chemoprophylaxis in developing countries. This was because it was so important that all available money should be used to cure infectious patients. However in recent years this opinion has altered a little, particularly with the coming of HIV infection and the AIDS epidemic. But **use each only in line with the recommendations of your National Tuberculosis Programme**.

Two terms are used to describe the two different types of preventive therapy.

1. **Preventive therapy** where a drug is given to individuals who have not been infected in order to prevent development of disease (e.g. infant being breast-fed; whole communities).
2. **Chemoprophylaxis** where the drug is used to prevent development of disease in people who have already been infected.

1: DRUGS

The drug which is used in chemoprophylaxis is **isoniazid**. It is used because it is cheap, has very few side-effects, can be taken by mouth – and has been proved to be effective. **Do not use rifampicin for chemoprophylaxis**. Isoniazid may not be effective in countries where there is a high level of primary drug resistance. The dose of isoniazid used is 5 mg/kg (not exceeding 300 mg) orally every day for a minimum of 6 months.

2: USE

If you decide to consider using either preventive therapy or chemoprophylaxis, remember that it is difficult enough to persuade people with tuberculosis to take treatment for a long time. How much more difficult it will be to persuade people who are well to take daily medicine for months, or give it to their children (see p 78). The following are **possible reasons for their use**. (In some of these you may not know whether or not the person has already been infected with TB. But the treatment is the same.)

1. patients infected with the human immunodeficiency virus (HIV) or suffering from AIDS.
2. breast-fed infants of sputum-positive mothers (p 165).
3. close contacts aged 5 years or under who have a strongly positive tuberculin test – an age group liable to suffer from tuberculous meningitis or miliary tuberculosis (p 77). See p 78 about explaining this treatment to parents. Above that age your National Programme may provide guidance.
4. newly-infected patients as shown by recent change in tuberculin test from negative to positive.
5. certain clinical states in which tuberculosis is more likely to develop e.g. Hodgkin's disease; prolonged treatment with prednisolone at a dose level exceeding 10 mg daily; leukaemia; anti-cancer drugs or severe diabetes mellitus. In a patient with chronic liver disease or in a heavy alcohol drinker, there is an increased risk of liver damage by isoniazid: only use if there is very good reason.
6. Controlled trials have shown that isoniazid chemoprophylaxis in HIV and tuberculin positive individuals reduces the risk of tuberculous disease. But WHO does not at present recommend its use, because funds are needed more urgently to treat actual patients. In some countries funds may be made available from AIDS programmes or elsewhere.

3: DOUBTFULLY ACTIVE TUBERCULOSIS

If you have a patient with a chest X-ray showing what seems to be a **doubtfully active tuberculous condition** do not give prophylaxis treatment with isoniazid. If you decide treatment is necessary, give full standard treatment (see p 165).

Appendix D
Infections with Opportunistic Mycobacteria

These are sometimes called 'atypical', 'anonymous' or 'mycobacteria other than tubercle bacilli'.

There are a number of different sorts of these bacteria. They are **common in water and soil** and associated with **various animals**.

They occasionally infect man and **cause chest disease like tuberculosis. Diagnosis** can only be made **by culture**.

Rarely, particularly in patients with AIDS, the bacteria spread through the bloodstream. They may then cause multiple bone abscesses etc.

In **countries with high prevalence of tuberculosis** these infections are **rare**, while tuberculosis is common. They will therefore not be important in your practice. In any case you need culture facilities to diagnose them. So we are only mentioning these infections briefly.

In countries where tuberculosis has greatly decreased, the frequency of infections with these bacteria has remained about the same. Most people easily control the infection and do not become ill. But AIDS patients have severely damaged defences. In Europe and America many AIDS patients die from these infections.

These bacteria are often **resistant** to some of the **usual drugs** used for treating tuberculosis. **Therefore only experienced specialists should treat these patients.**

Appendix E
Tuberculin Testing

First infection with the tubercle bacillus leads to the development of allergy to the protein tuberculin. When tuberculin is injected into the skin of an infected person a delayed local reaction develops in 24–48 hours. We list below conditions which may **depress this reaction**. The reaction measures the **degree of allergy**: it **does not measure immunity**. It does NOT indicate the presence or extent of disease.

A positive test only shows that the person has at some time been infected with TB. The proportion of people with positive tests will steadily increase with age. Many adults who are quite well will have positive tests.

Below we describe the material used in tuberculin testing and how to interpret the tests. In countries where HIV is a problem, remember the risk of spreading the infection. Use a separate syringe and needle (or Heaf gun blades) for each person.

1: TUBERCULINS

1.1 Recommended tuberculin

Internatonally WHO and the International Union Against Tuberculosis and Lung Disease recommend only using *PPD-RT23*. This is a purified tuberculin. In 1958 the State Serum Institute in Denmark prepared a very large batch for UNICEF and WHO. It is mixed with Tween 80 (a detergent to prevent the tuberculin sticking to the glass). It is used for tuberculin surveys throughout the world.

1.2 Storage

Keep tuberculin at a temperature not higher than 20°C, except for short periods when using it. Do not leave it in direct sunlight or strong daylight. Do not let it freeze. For storage the best temperature is 2–8°C. Do not keep used vials of tuberculin for more than 2 days.

2: TUBERCULIN TESTS

Only one test is now recommended by WHO and IUATLD: the Mantoux. In the British Isles the standard test is the Heaf, but it is little used elsewhere.

2.1 Mantoux test

(This section is based on the International Union Against Tuberculosis and Lung Disease recommendations: see Reference p 205).

2.1.1 The standard dose both for diagnostic work and for surveys is 2TU (Tuberculin Units) in 0.1 ml of PPD-RT23.

2.1.2 Choose an area of skin at the junction of the mid and upper thirds of the dorsal surface (back, more hairy) of the forearm. (This is WHO advice.) If you always choose the left arm, you will not be looking for the result on the wrong arm. Do not clean the arm with acetone or ether. If you use soap and water, see that the arm is dry before carrying out the test. In a struggling child ask a nurse or a relative to hold the arm gently but firmly.

2.1.3 Use the special disposable 1 ml syringe (graduated in 100ths of a ml). Use 26 gauge 10-mm long disposable needles with short bevel. (You can use 25 gauge if you cannot get 26 gauge.) Use a separate sterile syringe and needle for each person tested. Draw up a little more than 0.1 ml into the syringe. Hold it up and expel any air. Then adjust to exactly 0.1 ml by expelling extra solution.

2.1.4 Lightly stretch the skin. Insert the needle with the bevel upmost *into* (not under) the skin. Do not touch the plunger until the needle point is in the right place. Inject the exact volume of 0.1 ml. Remove your finger from the plunger before you withdraw the needle. This should produce a flat, pale weal with well-marked pits and a steep borderline.

If there is significant leakage of tuberculin (at the connection of needle and syringe or because the needle was not right in the skin) repeat the test more correctly on the other arm: make a special note of the arm with the good test so that you read the test on the correct arm.

Special Note on Tuberculin Tests for Diagnosis

Tuberculin PPD-RT23 is the standard international tuberculin for surveys. But it is very expensive. Many countries buy other cheaper, but standard, tuberculins. For diagnosis use a 2TU dose of the standard tuberculin provided in your own country. The method of injecting is as above.

2.2 Reading and interpreting the result

Read the test after 3–4 days. If a reaction has taken place you will see an area of erythema (redness) which may be difficult to see on a dark skin, and an area of induration (thickening) of the skin. You can feel the thickening even when

Mantoux tuberculin test

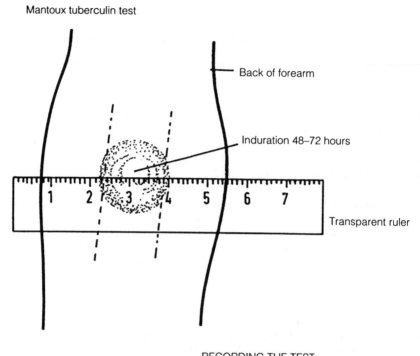

Back of forearm

Induration 48–72 hours

Transparent ruler

RECORDING THE TEST
1. Dose of tuberculin used (IU)
2. Time from test to reading it
3. Diameter of **induration** (not redness) in mm

Figure 35   *The Mantoux tuberculin test.* Record the horizontal width in mm of **induration** (the thickening of the skin, **not** the redness)

your eyes are closed. Measure the diameter of **induration** across the transverse axis of the arm (Figure 35). Record this diameter carefully, e.g. 'Mantoux 12 mm'.

The amount of erythema (redness) present is not important.

In this book we are only concerned with using the tuberculin reaction to help in diagnosis. For this you can record a **positive** reaction as an area of induration of the skin with a diameter of 10 mm or above. But record the measured diameter of the induration also. Above 10 mm diameter, the bigger the size of the reaction the more positive is the test. If the diameter is below 10 mm it is not definitely positive. But remember that malnutrition or severe illness, among other things (p 203), can make the test less positive. For a particular patient you will have to consider the result of the test together with **all** the other information about that patient.

The more positive the test, the more important it is as evidence that you may be dealing with a case of tuberculosis. **But** remember that it is only **one point** in favour of the diagnosis. Many well people have a strongly positive test. However a strongly positive test is a particularly valuable point in a child, especially a very young child.

On the other hand a **negative test does not exclude tuberculosis**. A patient with active tuberculosis may have the tuberculin test **suppressed** by a number of factors e.g. malnutrition, viral infections, HIV infection, measles, chickenpox, glandular fever, cancer, severe bacteriological infections (including tuberculosis), corticosteroids and similar drugs.

A positive result is usual after previous **BCG vaccination**, at least for a number of years. But this is usually a weaker reaction, often with a diameter less than 10 mm.

3: HEAF TEST

In this test you use a simple instrument – a Heaf gun. It consists of six spring-loaded needles which when fired pierce the skin through a drop of undiluted PPD. (One advantage is that undiluted PPD lasts indefinitely.) Use the 'magnetic' Heaf gun with disposable blades. Discard the blades after each test to avoid the risk of spreading HIV.

3.1   Method

Using a dropper, place a drop of undiluted PPD on the clean dry skin at the junction of the mid and upper third of the anterior (front, smooth-skinned) surface of the left forearm.

1. Adjust the length of the needles (2 mm for adults, 1 mm for young children).
2. Dip the end-plate and needles of the gun into a shallow dish containing spirit and ignite them in the flame of a spirit lamp.
3. Cool for not less than 10 seconds.
4. Place the end-plate firmly over the drop of tuberculin.
5. Depress the handle of the gun thus causing the needles to pierce the skin.

DO NOT PRODUCE A BURN ON THE SKIN

3.2   Reading the test (Figure 36)

You should read the test at 48–72 hours though it may still be possible to read a strong reaction for 7 days or more after the test. Record the result as one of the four grades given below:

Grade 0	No reaction.
Grade I	Palpable induration (papule) around at least four puncture points.
Grade II	Papules have formed a ring.
Grade III	A solid area of induration has been formed.

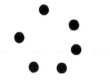

Grade I. Palpable reaction around at least 4 needle points

Grade II. The papules are larger and have joined to form a ring

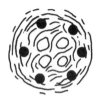

Grade III. The papules are larger still and have filled in the centre

Grade IV. There is a large thick plaque (raised area), larger than the end-plate of the gun. There are vesicles (blebs) in the centre of the plaque

Figure 36   *Grades of reaction to the Heaf test*

Grade IV   There are shiny vesicles over the solid area. There may be surrounding erythema (redness).

There is general agreement that Grades II, III and IV indicate a 'positive' reaction. Record the Grade carefully.

4: INTERPRETING A TUBERCULIN TEST

We can summarise this as follows:

4.1 Epidemiology

If you are using the test for epidemiology (to measure the number of **infected** people in the community) there is probably a national rule about what is regarded as positive. You should follow this. It will recommend that you record the diameter of the induration for each test. Positives will probably include a diameter of 10 mm or more to the doses in the Mantoux test given above **or** Grade II, III or IV on the Heaf test. But WHO recommends that the Heaf test should not be used for epidemiological surveys.

4.2 Diagnosis

If you are using the test as a help in diagnosis the problem is more difficult:

1. A diameter of induration of **less than 10 mm** should be graded 'negative'. This does NOT EXCLUDE A DIAGNOSIS OF TUBERCULOSIS. The reaction may be suppressed by malnutrition, other conditions (see p 203, paragraph 2.2) or by the severity of the tuberculosis.
2. A diameter of **10 mm or more** in a child or adult who has **not had BCG** (look for scar) is **positive**. A diameter of **over 15 mm** in a child who **has had BCG** is **positive** (smaller reactions could be due to the BCG): this means the child has also been infected with TB.

The larger the diameter (above 10–15 mm) the greater the support for a diagnosis of tuberculosis.
   The younger the child the stronger is this support.

Reference

Arnadottir T., Rieder H.L., Trébucq A., Waaler H.T. Guidelines for conducting tuberculin skin test surveys in high prevalence countries. *Tubercle and Lung Disease* 1996: **77** (Suppl.): 1–20.

Appendix F
Gastric Suction in Children

In adults the diagnosis of pulmonary tuberculosis depends on finding TB in the sputum. But children under the age of 10 years swallow their sputum. They find it difficult to produce a specimen for examination.

When you cannot obtain sputum the only effective method is gastric suction. The method is distressing to the child. Only use it when you can culture the specimen for TB. Only use it when there is a particularly difficult clinical problem. If you do use it, pay particular attention to the following detail.

It is best to get the specimen of stomach contents first thing in the morning before the child has had anything to eat or drink. Pass a soft rubber tube or catheter into the stomach. Then suck the contents into a large syringe. The amount will vary from a few ml to about 50 ml. If the tube blocks while sucking, inject a few ml of water (less than 20 ml). If that is necessary, wait a few minutes. Then suck again with the syringe. Place the material in a container with buffer fluid (sodium hydrogen phosphate). If mucus or mucopus rises to the surface, remove it and stain for TB. Culture it also for TB. If nothing rises to the surface, allow the fluid to stand for 24 hours. Stand it in the dark: sunlight will kill the bacilli. The material will sink to the bottom of the container. Then stain this for TB and send for culture.

Glossary

The glossary is to explain some of the words used in the book. It is particularly for readers who are not doctors and those who are not yet very fluent in the English language. Words often have more than one meaning. **Here we only explain the meaning used in this book.**

ABBREVIATION: A shortened way of stating something, e.g. 'S' as short for 'streptomycin'.

ABDUCTION: Outward (sideways) movement, usually of the leg.

ABNORMAL: Not normal.

ABSCESS: A local collection of pus.

ACETABULUM: The socket of the hip joint.

ADHESIONS: Things sticking together.

ADJACENT: Close to, beside.

ADMINISTER: Give a drug or a treatment.

ADVERSE: Bad, harmful.

AGRANULOCYTOSIS: Absence of the polymorph white blood cells.

AIDS: Acquired ImmunoDeficiency Syndrome: A chronic fatal illness due to HIV (see glossary). The virus destroys immune cells. The patient gets a series of other infections as his defences are weakened. Tuberculosis is commonly one of those infections.

AMENORRHOEA: Absence of the female periods.

AMOEBIC ABSCESS: A local collection of pus due to *Entamoeba histolytica*, an amoeba causing dysentry. The infection may spread from the bowel to the liver, causing an abscess.

ANAPHYLAXIS: Sudden collapse due to allergy (hypersensitivity).

ANEURYSM: Local dilatation of the aorta, or other artery, due to disease.

ANOREXIA: Having no appetite for food.

ANTERIOR: In the front. The front part.

APLASTIC ANAEMIA: A type of anaemia in which the normal blood cells do not get formed.

ANTICONVULSANT: Drug to stop fits in epilepsy.

ARACHNOIDITIS: Inflammation of the membranes of the spinal cord.

ARTHRALGIA: Pain in the joints.

ASCITES: Fluid in the peritoneal cavity.

ASPIRATION: Drawing in, e.g. breath into the lungs or fluid into a syringe.

ASPHYXIA: Death from sudden cutting off of the air to the lungs.

ATAXIA: Unsteadiness when walking.

ATROPHY: Wasting away (of an organ of the body).

AXILLA: Armpit.

BACILLI: Bacteria looking like little rods.

BACTERICIDAL: Killing the bacteria.

BACTERIOSTATIC: Stopping bacteria growing (but not actually killing them).

BCG: Bacille Calmette-Guérin. A vaccine against tuberculosis developed by two French doctors, Calmette and Guérin.

BILIRUBIN: A pigment in the bile.

BIOPSY: Cutting out a small area of tissue to examine under the microscope. This is done to try to make the diagnosis.

BROAD SPECTRUM (of an antibiotic): A drug which kills a wide range of bacteria.

BRONCHIECTASIS: Widening of the tubes of the bronchi due to damage to their walls by disease.

BRONCHOSCOPY: Visual examination of the inside of the bronchi through a bronchoscope.

BRONCHUS, BRONCHI: Tube, tubes, through which the air goes in and out of the lungs.

BURKITT'S LYMPHOMA: A cancer of upper or lower jaw which occurs particularly in children in tropical Africa.

CALCIFICATION: Laying down of calcium. This is usually visible as areas of marked whiteness in the X-ray.

CANDIDA INFECTION: A fungus infection. Usually produces white painful patches, often in the mouth.

CARCINOMA: A cancer.

CASEATION: The breakdown of tissue killed by tubercle bacilli into a yellow cheese-like material (which, in the lungs, may later turn into liquid and be coughed up).

CASE-FINDING: Discovering patients (in this case with tuberculosis).

CAVITY: A hole in a tissue. In the lung it usually contains air. In the kidney it usually contains caseous material.

CERVICAL: In the neck.

CHEMOPROPHYLAXIS: Giving a drug or drugs to prevent disease.

CHEMOTHERAPY: Treatment with chemical drugs (though this includes, in tuberculosis, antibiotics like streptomycin).

CHOROIDAL TUBERCLES: Tubercles (see glossary) of the choroid membrane at the back of the eye. These can be seen through an ophthalmoscope.

'CLASSICAL': Here means 'the usual form described in the text books'.

COLD ABSCESS: A collection of pus, or fluid caseous material, due to tuberculosis. It is **not** hot, red and tender like a septic abscess, so it is called 'cold'. It may slowly break through the skin to the surface.

COMA: Continuous unconsciousness.

COMPLICATION: Secondary or later damage (sometimes in other organs) due to a lesion or a disease. A disease resulting from another disease.

COMPLEX: Two or more things which go together or are connected. See 'Primary Complex'.

COMPLIANCE: The patient obeying, and sticking to, the advice given.

COMPONENT: Part of something.

CONGENITAL: Inherited from one or both parents.

CONFLUENT: Running or flowing together.

CONJUNCTIVA: The membrane over the front of the eye and the inner surface of the eyelids.

CONSTRICTIVE: Holding tightly, squeezing.

CONTACTS: People, often members of the family, who have been close to the patient and whom he might have infected.

CORNEA: The clear surface of the eyeball lying in front of the pupil.

CORTEX: The outer part (of the brain or kidney).

CORTICOSTEROID DRUGS: Drugs which suppress (decrease) inflammation. They also decrease the body's defences.

CREPITATIONS: Moist sounds coming from small amounts of fluid in the lungs. These make a crackling noise (heard through the stethoscope) when the patient breathes in.

CRITERIA: Reasons or facts, e.g. the criteria or reasons for making a particular diagnosis such as tuberculosis.

CRYPTIC: Hidden, obscure. Applied to a type of miliary tuberculosis difficult to diagnose.

CSF: Cerebrospinal fluid.

CYANOSIS: The patient looking blue due to lack of oxygen.

CYSTITIS: Inflammation of the bladder.

CUTANEOUS: Of the skin.

DEFAULT: Patient stopping coming for treatment.

DERMATITIS: Inflammation of the skin.

DERIVATIVE: Something derived or got out of something.

DESENSITISATION: Method for curing hypersensitivity in a patient.

DISC (VERTEBRAL): Rounded discs (flattened circles) of cartilage between the vertebrae.

DISCHARGE: Material, such as fluid or pus, pushed out from a lesion, often through the skin.

DISSEMINATED: Arising in many different organs in the body. The infection or disease usually gets there through the bloodstream.

DONOR: Someone who gives blood for transfusion.

DORMANT: Sleeping or inactive. Applied to a tuberculous lesion or tubercle bacilli.

ECTOPIC PREGNANCY: A pregnancy in which the fetus begins to develop outside the uterus (womb) in a fallopian tube.

ECZEMA: A chronic itching rash.

EMBOLISM: A clot which travels through the bloodstream and finally blocks a blood vessel. This usually cuts off its blood flow.

EMPYEMA: Pus in the space between the layer of pleura covering the lung and the layer of pleura covering the inner side of the chest wall.

ENDOCRINE: Chemicals controlling body function produced by endocrine glands e.g. adrenals.

ENDOMETRIUM: The mucous membrane lining the inside of the uterus.

ENTERIC: A word often used for typhoid or paratyphoid.

ENVIRONMENT: The surroundings in which people live.

EPIDIDYMIS: An organ lying above and behind the testis. It consists of little tubes leading to a densely folded tube which carries the sperm to the spermatic cord.

EPIGLOTTIS: The firm flap at the back of the tongue which prevents food getting into the larynx and trachea when you swallow.

EROSION: Wearing away.

ERYTHEMA: Redness.

EXTRA-PULMONARY DISEASE: Disease outside the lungs, in other organs of the body.

EXUDATE: Fluid and inflammatory cells in an area of disease.

FALLOPIAN TUBES: The tubes down which the ovum (egg) is carried from the ovary to the uterus (womb).

FETAL: Of or in the unborn baby.

FETUS: Unborn baby.

FIBROSIS: Scar tissue, especially in the lung.

FISTULA: A connection between an inflammatory lesion in tissue or bone and the skin. It usually discharges pus. **Or** an abnormal connection (due to disease) between two cavities in the body, e.g. between bladder and rectum.

FLUCTUANT: An area of disease which contains fluid which can be moved by pressing with the fingers.

FLUOROSCOPY: A special dye on the TB gives out light when ultraviolet light is shone on the slide under the microscope. The TB show as small spots of light against the dark background.

FOCUS, usually 'primary focus': The changes in an organ due to the first infection with tubercle bacilli.

FORMULATION: The form in which the drug or drugs are prepared for the patient.

GASTRIC SUCTION OR LAVAGE: Removal of stomach contents, sometimes after injecting saline. The patient first swallows a rubber tube. The fluid is then sucked out with a syringe.

GASTRO-INTESTINAL: To do with the stomach and intestines.

GIBBUS: An acute angle in the spine due to collapse of a vertebra from disease.

GYNAECOMASTIA: Swelling of the male breasts.

HAEMATOGENOUS: Carried through the bloodstream.

HAEMOLYTIC ANAEMIA: Anaemia in which the red blood cells are destroyed.

HAEMOPTYSIS: Coughing up blood.

HEPATITIS: Inflammation of the liver.

HEPATOTOXIC: Damage to the liver.

HERPES ZOSTER: A virus infection of the nerve roots. Produces pain in the area supplied by the nerve, with a skin rash in the same area.

HILAR: At the root of the lung.

HILUM: The root of the lung.

HISTOLOGY: Examining tissue under the miscroscope.

HIV: Human ImmunoDeficiency Virus, the cause of AIDS (see glossary).

HYDROCEPHALUS: Literally 'water in the brain'. Enlargement of the ventricles (internal spaces of the brain). Usually due to obstruction to the circulation of the brain fluid (cerebrospinal fluid or 'CSF').

HYGIENE: Actions to make people's surroundings (environment) more healthy.

HYPERPLASTIC: With much inflammatory tissue (producing a lump or mass).

HYPERSENSITIVITY: Reactions in certain patients caused by even small doses of a drug or other substance (e.g. tuberculin). These doses have no harmful effect in normal people.

HYPOKALAEMIA: Low blood potassium.

HYPOTHYROIDISM: Decrease of the secretions of the thyroid gland leading to slowness of activity etc.

IMMUNISATION: Building up a person's defences against a disease, usually by giving a vaccine.

IMMUNOSUPPRESSANT DRUGS: Drugs which suppress the normal defences (immunity) of the body. Example: corticosteroid drugs.

INCIDENCE: The rate of new cases of a disease in a given time (usually a year).

INDURATION: Thickening. Usually in describing skin, e.g in the tuberculin test.

INFARCTION: Damage to a local area of tissue caused by a blocked blood vessel (usually blocked by a clot).

INFERIOR: Below. The lower part.

INFERTILE: Unable to produce babies.

INDURATION: Thickening.

INGUINAL LIGAMENT: The ligament across the groin.

INHALATION: Breathing something in.

INTERMITTENT: Less than daily, e.g. twice weekly.

INTRAMUSCULAR: Into the muscle.

INTRATHECAL: Into the spinal fluid.

INTRATHORACIC: Inside the chest.

INTRAVENOUS: Into a vein.

LACHRYMATION: Tears from the eye(s).

LARYNGEAL SWAB: A swab of cotton wool on a stick which is passed into the larynx to take a specimen to examine for TB.

LATENT: Something that is there but not obvious; it can later become obvious.

LESION: An area of disease in the body.

LEUCOPENIA: Decrease in numbers of the white blood cells.

LEUKAEMIA: A cancer of the white blood cells.

LOCALISED: A diseased area only in a small part of a tissue of the body.

LUMBAR: The lower part of the back.

LUMEN: The space in the middle, e.g. the part of the bronchus containing the air.

LUPOID: Like lupus. See Lupus Vulgaris: Text p 132.

LYMPHADENOMA: One kind of cancer of the lymph nodes.

LYMPH NODES: Rounded or oval lumps of lymph tissue. The lymph flows through them. They play a part in the body's defences. When enlarged they can be felt in the neck, groin or armpit. There are also many in the mediastinum and in the abdomen. They are often affected by tuberculosis. Some people still call them 'lymph glands'.

LYMPHOMA: Usually tumour of lymph nodes. But Burkitt's lymphoma (see glossary) usually arises in the jaw.

MALAISE: Feeling ill.

MALNUTRITION: Not having enough food, or enough of the right sorts of food.

MASS TREATMENT: Treating large numbers of patients.

MASTOID PROCESS: Part of the skull behind the ear. The inside part may get infected from the ear.

MEDIASTINUM: The central area in the chest behind the breastbone (sternum) and between the two lungs. It contains the heart, great vessels, trachea, oesophagus (gullet) and lymph nodes.

MENINGITIS: Inflammation of the membranes covering the brain.

MICROSCOPY: Examining through a microscope.

MILIARY TUBERCULOSIS: Small areas of tuberculosis spread by the blood-stream into many organs of the body. 'Miliary' because pathologists thought they looked like millet seeds.

MUTANT: A bacillus which has suddenly changed and become different from the rest of the population. It will then pass on the change to its descendants. Here the change is to drug-resistance.

MYOCARDIUM: Muscle of the heart.

NAUSEA: Feeling of sickness, feeling like vomiting.

NECROTIC: Tissue completely broken down by disease. Dead tissue.

NEUROPATHY: Damage to the nerves. Peripheral neuropathy: damage to the nerves of the limbs.

NODULAR: Lumpy.

NON-REACTIVE: Not producing the usual microscopic picture of tuberculosis.

NOURISHED: Well-nourished: well-fed. Malnourished: not enough food.

NUTRITION, state of: Whether the person has had enough food. Malnutrition: Not having enough food.

NYSTAGMUS: Quick, regular, horizontal eye movements when a patient is asked to fix his eyes on an object to one side. It is not normal.

OEDEMA: Abnormal increase of body fluid in a tissue.

OPHTHALMOSCOPE: An instrument for examining the retina of the eye.

OPPORTUNISTIC MYCOBACTERIA: Bacteria like tubercle bacilli which exist in the environment and may sometimes 'take the opportunity' to invade and damage man, especially when his defences are reduced, e.g. by HIV infection. In normal people the body's defences prevent them causing damage.

ORAL: By the mouth.

OTOTOXICITY: Damage to the ears.

PANCYTOPENIA: Decrease in the numbers of all kinds of blood cells.

PANOPHTHALMITIS: Inflammation of the whole of the eye.

PAPILLOEDEMA: Blurring of the retina round the optic nerve due to back pressure. (As seen through the ophthalmoscope.)

PARAPLEGIA: Paralysis of the legs.

PARATRACHEAL: Beside the trachea.

PARTURITION: Birth of the baby from the mother.

PATHOGENESIS: How a disease arises. PATHOGENIC: Giving rise to disease. NON-PATHOGENIC: **Not** giving rise to disease.

PELVIS (of kidney): The root of the kidney where the urine gathers before passing on into the ureter.

PERICARDIUM: The membranes round the heart.

PERITONEUM: The membrane covering the intestine and the wall of the cavity in which the intestine lies.

PHOTOPHOBIA: Discomfort when looking at light.

PIGMENTATION: Dark colour (of the skin or mucous membrane).

PLEURA: The membrane covering the lung and the wall of the chest cavity containing the lung.

PLACENTA: The tissue full of blood vessels between the fetus (unborn child) and the wall of the uterus (womb).

PNEUMOTHORAX: Air in the pleural space between the lung and the chest wall.

POLYMORPH WHITE BLOOD CELLS: Cells with lobed nuclei (the densely staining centre part of the cell).

POSTERIOR: At the back. The back part.

POSTMORTEM EXAMINATION: Examination of a dead body by a pathologist.

POST-PRIMARY LESION OF TUBERCULOSIS: The changes in the body caused by the later stages of the disease **after** those of primary tuberculosis.

PREVALENCE: The proportion of people in a community with a particular disease (e.g. tuberculosis) at any one time.

PRIMARY COMPLEX: The tuberculous lesion in an organ after the first infection **together with** the tuberculous lesions in the draining lymph nodes.

PRIMARY LESION: The changes in an organ due to the first infection with tubercle bacilli. Often called the 'primary focus'.

PRIMARY TUBERCULOSIS: The lesions produced by a first (new) infection with tuberculosis.

PROGRESSION, PROGRESSIVE: Getting worse.

PROGNOSIS: What will happen to the disease (and the patient), e.g. getting better or worse.

PRONATE: Turn the hand with palm (front) downwards.

PROPHYLAXIS: Prevention of disease in a person.

PROSPECTIVE, of a trial: Here a trial in which the researchers give BCG to a large group of people. They then follow the group for number of years to see how many develop tuberculosis, compared with an unvaccinated group.

PROSTATE: A gland surrounding the male urethra (the tube which carries the urine away from the bladder). The prostate lies just in front of the rectum. It adds fluids to the semen (the fluid which carries the sperm).

PSOAS ABSCESS: A cold abscess showing just below the groin. The tuberculous pus comes from disease of the spine. The pus makes its way down the covering of the psoas muscle to the groin.

PURPURA: Blotches of blood under the skin.

PURULENT: Containing pus.

PYOGENIC: Bacteria which cause pus.

PYOPNEUMOTHORAX: Pus and air together in the pleural space.

PYRAMID (of kidney): The middle part of the kidney between the root (pelvis) and the other part (cortex).

PYREXIA: Fever, raised body temperature.

RADIOLOGICAL: By X-ray.

REACTIVATION: Disease which had become inactive (dormant) but starting to get active again.

REGIMEN: A drug, or group of drugs, given together for a stated time.

RELAPSE: Disease starting again after it had seemed to be cured.

RENAL: Of the kidney.

RESECT: Remove by surgery.

RESEMBLES: Looks like.

RETROBULBAR NEURITIS: Inflammation of the optic nerve behind the eye.

RETROGRADE: Backwards or from below.

RHONCHI: Wheezing noises which come from the bronchi and are heard through the stethoscope. They are due to narrowing of the bronchi by fluid, swelling or contraction.

SECONDARY DEPOSIT: A new area of cancer somewhere in the body arising from cells from a primary (first) cancer carried by the blood or lymph.

SEMINAL VESICLES: Sacs about 5 cm long which lie above the prostate on each side and in front of the rectum. They produce part of the semen.

SENSITIVITY TESTS: Tests of tubercle bacilli (TB) for sensitivity or resistance to anti-tuberculosis drugs.

SEPTIC: With pus.

SHOCK: Collapse with lowered blood pressure.

SINUS: A connection between a lesion and the surface, usually through the skin.

SPECTRUM: See 'Broad Spectrum'.

SPINAL BLOCK: An obstruction to the normal flow of cerebrospinal fluid along the spinal cord.

SPUTUM: Spit.

STERILISE: Kill off all bacteria, viruses etc., e.g. by heating.

STERILISATION: The process of sterilising.

SUBSEQUENTLY: Afterwards, later.

SUBSTITUTE: Give instead of.

SUPERFICIAL: Near or on the surface.

SUPERIOR: Above. The upper part.

SUPERVISION: Watching closely over.

SURVEILLANCE: Watching over the patient and his progress under treatment.

SYNOVIUM: The tissue enclosing a joint.

SYNDROME: A group of symptoms and signs.

TB: Tubercle bacilli.

THORAX: The chest.

THORACIC: Of the chest.

THRUSH: Fungus infection of mouth with painful white patches.

THROMBOCYTOPENIA: Decrease in the platelets of the blood. These are essential for clotting of the blood to stop bleeding.

TINNITUS: Ringing or buzzing in the ears.

TOLERATE (of a drug): Take without any trouble.

TOXICITY: Poisoning or damaging effects, e.g. of medicines.

TRACHEA: The windpipe connecting the larynx to the bronchi.

TUBERCLES: Small rounded areas of tuberculous disease. These gave the disease its name.

TUBERCULIN: Protein extracted from tubercle bacilli. The infected person becomes sensitive to this protein, as shown by tuberculin skin tests.

TUBERCULOMA: A rounded area of disease, usually 1 cm or more in diameter.

TYPHOID: An acute bacterial disease which produces fever and intestinal symptoms. Sometimes called 'enteric'.

URETER: The tube carrying urine from the kidney to the bladder.

UVEITIS: Inflammation of the part of the eyeball which includes the iris, ciliary body and choroid.

VARIANT: Different sort, alternative.

VERTIGO: Giddiness.

WASTING, usually of muscles: Muscles smaller than on the other side.

References

The following are useful publications. They can be obtained from the addresses indicated.

World Health Organization (WHO). Global Tuberculosis Programme. 1211 Geneva 27, Switzerland, or through Regional Offices of WHO

1. Maher, D., Chaulet, P., Spinaci, S., Harries, A. *Treatment of Tuberculosis: Guidelines for National Programmes*. 2nd edn. Geneva: WHO, 1997.
2. Harries, A.D., Maher, D. *TB/HIV. A Clinical Manual*. Geneva: WHO, 1996. Obtainable from TALC at a cheaper rate. A very useful manual. It also covers other complications of AIDS which may occur in your tuberculosis patients.
3. *Tuberculosis Control Handbook*. Geneva: WHO, Forthcoming. A reference book on the subject.
4. *Technical Guidelines for Tuberculosis Control*. New Delhi, India: Directorate General of Health Services, 1997. A recent example of the outline of a National Programme.
5. Crofton, J., Chaulet, P., Maher, D. *Guidelines for the Management of Drug-resistant Tuberculosis*. Geneva: WHO, 1997. A technical guide for specialist centres managing these difficult cases.
6. WHO Global Programme on AIDS. *Counselling for HIV/AIDS: a key to caring*. Geneva: WHO, 1995.
7. WHO Global Programme on AIDS. *AIDS Homecare Handbook*. Geneva: WHO, 1993.
8. WHO Global Programme on AIDS. *AIDS in Africa. A Manual for Physicians*. Geneva: WHO, 1992.
9. WHO Global Programme on AIDS. *Management of Sexually Transmitted Diseases*. Geneva: WHO, 1994.

International Union Against Tuberculosis and Lung Disease (IUALTD): 68 boulevard Saint-Michel, 75006 Paris, France

10. Enarson, D.A., Rieder, H.L., Arnadottir, T., Trebucq, A. *Tuberculosis Guide for Low Income Countries*. 4th edn. Paris: IUATLD, 1996. An excellent short guide to tuberculosis control.
11. IUATLD. *Technical Guide for Sputum Examination by Direct Microscopy*. Paris:

IUATLD, 1978. A very useful practice guide, particularly designed for developing countries.

TALC: Teaching Aids at Low Cost. PO Box 49, St Albans, Herts AL1 4AX, UK

A non-profit making organisation set up to supply books, slides and other materials for the training of health workers. Free list of books and material obtainable at the above address. Further copies of the low cost edition of *Clinical Tuberculosis* are also available for despatch from TALC. Reduced rate for multiple copies. Some WHO publications (e.g. References 1 and 2) are also supplied at low cost.

12. Dean, P., Ebrahim, G.J. *The Practical Care of Sick Children. A Manual for Use in Small Tropical Hospitals*. London: Macmillan, 1986. ISBN 0–333–42347–X.
13. Werner, D. *Where There is No Doctor*. Highly practical. Many illustrations. International version or African version (illustrations and traditional treatments vary). Also Portuguese and Spanish translations. Widely used internationally.
14. King, F.S., Burgess, A. *Nutrition for Developing Countries*. Particular reference to children.
15. Bever, M., Ray, S. *Women and HIV/AIDS*. Impact of HIV/AIDS on women's health, sexual relations and reproductive rights. What women round the world are doing about it.
16. Two sets of 24 teaching slides
    a) *Natural History of Childhood Tuberculosis*
    b) *Pathology of Tuberculosis in Children. Macroscopic and microscopic.*

Other fuller texts

17. Davies, P.D.O. (ed.) *Clinical Tuberculosis*. 2nd edn. London: Chapman and Hall, 1998. A comprehensive international multi-author reference book on all aspects of tuberculosis, including control in high prevalence countries.
18. Seaton, A., Seaton, D., Leitch, A.G. *Crofton and Douglas's Respiratory Diseases*. 4th edn. Oxford: Blackwell Scientific, 1989. 5th edn: Forthcoming. Includes a detailed postgraduate text on the epidemiology and pulmonary aspects of tuberculosis.
19. Miller, F.J.W. *Tuberculosis in Children*. New Delhi, India: Churchill-Livingstone, 1986. ISBN 81–7042–0010. A short text describing the natural history, epidemiology and clinical investigation of tuberculosis in children in regions of high and low infection and morbidity.
20. Ryan, F. *Tuberculosis. The Greatest Story Never Told*. Bromsgrove, England: Swift, 1992. ISBN 81–874082–00–6. A fascinating history of the research and personalities leading to the modern chemotherapy of the disease.

Other Macmillan
Health Titles

Care of the Critically Ill Patient in the Tropics and Subtropics: D. Watters, I. Wilson, R. Leaver and A. Bagshawe 0–333–53799–8
Common Medical Problems in the Tropics Revised Edition: C.R. Schull 0–333–67999–7
Communicating Health: J. Hubley 0–333–57679–9
Immunization in Practice: WHO 0–333–63095–5
Paediatric Practice: G.J. Ebrahim 0–333–57347–1
Practical Care of Sick Children: P. Dean and G.J. Ebrahim 0–333–42347–X
Refugee Health: Medécins Sans Frontiéres 0–333–72210–8
Setting Up Community Health Programmes: E. Lankaster 0–333–57423–0
Where There is No Doctor: D. Werner (Hesperian Foundation) 0–333–51651–6
Where Women Have No Doctor: A. August Burns, Ronnie Lovich, Jane Maxwell, Katherine Chapiro (Hesperian Foundation) 0–333–64933–8

Index